Table of Conte

Introduction

Welcome to "Smoothie Sensations: Blending Health and Flavor," a vibrant journey through the world of smoothies, tailored especially for the American palate. This book is more than just a collection of recipes; it's an exploration of how simple, fresh ingredients can transform into delicious and nutritious beverages.

Smoothies are not only a quick and convenient way to boost your intake of fruits, vegetables, and other essential nutrients, but they also offer an array of health benefits. They can be a powerful tool for weight management, a reliable source of energy, and a perfect option for on-the-go meals or snacks. The versatility of smoothies means they can be adapted to suit any taste or dietary need, making them a fantastic addition to any lifestyle.

Whether you're a fitness enthusiast looking for a protein-packed post-workout treat, a busy professional seeking a speedy yet healthy breakfast alternative, or someone exploring ways to incorporate more fruits and vegetables into your diet, smoothies are the answer. They are a delightful way to consume a concentrated dose of vitamins, minerals, and antioxidants, which can enhance your overall health, improve digestion, and even boost your immune system.

Our recipes range from classic and beloved flavors to innovative combinations that will tantalize your taste buds. Each recipe is crafted with the American flavor profile in mind, ensuring that every sip is both familiar and exciting. Moreover, we've included tips on how to customize your smoothies, making them perfect for any time of day and any dietary preference.

So, grab your blender, and let's embark on this flavorful journey together, where health meets taste in every glass!

This introduction sets the tone for a smoothie recipe book that emphasizes health benefits, convenience, and adaptability, appealing to a wide range of American readers.

CHAPTER 1

The Basics of Smoothie Making
Introduction to Techniques and Tips for the Perfect Smoothie

Welcome to the exciting world of smoothie making! This section serves as your guide to mastering the art of creating the perfect smoothie. Whether you're a beginner or a seasoned smoothie enthusiast, understanding the basics is key to crafting delicious, nutritious blends that cater to your taste and health goals.

1. Choosing the Right Ingredients:

- *Fruits and Vegetables:* The backbone of any smoothie, choose fresh or frozen fruits and vegetables. Frozen fruits can provide a thicker texture.
- *Liquids:* Your choice of liquid (milk, almond milk, coconut water, juice, or plain water) can significantly affect the taste and consistency of your smoothie.
- *Proteins:* Add protein powders, Greek yogurt, or nut butter for a protein boost, especially useful for meal replacement or post-workout smoothies.
- *Sweeteners:* Opt for natural sweeteners like honey, agave nectar, or ripe bananas. Remember, many fruits already add natural sweetness.
- *Superfoods and Supplements:* Chia seeds, flaxseeds, spirulina, or acai powder can add nutritional value to your smoothie.

2. Understanding Equipment:

- *Blenders:* A high-quality blender is crucial for a smooth, well-blended smoothie. High-speed blenders are best for breaking down ingredients like frozen fruits and nuts.
- *Measuring Tools:* Use measuring cups and spoons for consistent results, especially when experimenting with new recipes.
- *Glassware and Straws:* Choose the right glassware for serving, and consider reusable straws for an eco-friendly option.

3. Mastering the Technique:

- **Layering Ingredients:** Start with liquids, followed by softer ingredients (like fresh fruits), and add harder or frozen ingredients last. This helps in blending smoothly.
- **Balancing Flavors:** Experiment with different combinations to find what you enjoy. Balancing sweetness with a touch of acidity (like lemon or lime) can enhance flavors.
- **Texture**: Adjust the thickness by adding more liquid or using ingredients like banana or yogurt to thicken your smoothie.

4. Serving and Enjoyment:

- *Temperature:* Serve your smoothie immediately for the best taste and texture. Use ice or frozen fruits for a chilled smoothie.
- *Presentation:* Garnish with a slice of fruit, a sprinkle of seeds, or a dash of cinnamon for visual appeal.

5. Storing Leftovers:

- *Refrigeration:* Store any leftover smoothie in the refrigerator and consume it within 24 hours for the best quality.
- *Freezing:* You can freeze smoothies in ice cube trays and blend them again when needed.

Understanding these basics will set the foundation for your smoothie-making journey. Remember, the beauty of smoothies lies in their versatility and the ability to customize according to your preferences and nutritional needs. Let your creativity flow and start blending your way to delicious health!

The Ultimate Guide to Smoothie-Making Tools and Ingredients

Welcome to the section where we explore the essential tools and the finest ingredients that make for an unparalleled smoothie-making experience. In this guide, we'll dive into the world of blenders, superfoods, and specialty ingredients, ensuring that you are well-equipped to create smoothies that are not just delicious but also packed with nutrition.

Blenders: Your Key to the Perfect Smoothie

High-End Blenders:

- *Vitamix Series:* Known for their power and durability, Vitamix blenders are a top choice for smoothie aficionados. Ideal for those who use their blender daily and appreciate a range of textures.
- *Blendtec Models:* Blendtec offers a series of blenders with strong motors and unique blending cycles, perfect for those who enjoy tech-friendly features.
- *Breville Super Blenders:* Breville blenders combine style with functionality, offering pre-set functions for various blends.

Mid-Range Options:

- ***Ninja Professional Blenders:*** Ninja blenders provide excellent value, combining powerful blending capabilities with more affordable pricing.
- ***NutriBullet Series:*** Compact and convenient, NutriBullets are great for single servings and small kitchens, without compromising on the blending power.

Budget-Friendly Choices:

- ***Hamilton Beach Blenders:*** These blenders are perfect for occasional users who need a reliable appliance without a hefty price tag.
- **Oster Blenders:** Oster offers a range of affordable blenders that are suitable for basic smoothie recipes.

Superfoods and Organic Produce: Elevating Your Smoothie Game

- **Superfoods:** Look for organic and sustainably sourced superfoods like chia seeds, flaxseeds, hemp seeds, acai powder, spirulina, and matcha. Health food stores and online platforms like Amazon, Thrive Market, and iHerb offer a wide variety of these nutrient-packed ingredients.
- **Organic Produce:** Organic fruits and vegetables are crucial for a clean and healthy smoothie. Shop at local farmers' markets, join a Community Supported Agriculture (CSA) program or check out organic sections in grocery stores.

For exotic or off-season items, specialty grocery stores or online retailers can be excellent sources.

Unique Ingredients for Adventurous Blends

Explore specialty health food stores or ethnic markets for unique ingredients like dragon fruit, jackfruit, guava, or taro. Online stores like Exotic Fruit Market or Melissa's Produce offer a wide range of unusual fruits and vegetables that can add an exciting twist to your smoothies.

Measurement Equivalents

Liquid Measurements:

Cups to Milliliters (mL) and Liters (L):
- 1 cup = 240 mL
- 1/2 cup = 120 mL
- 1/3 cup = 80 mL
- 1/4 cup = 60 mL
- 1 tablespoon (Tbsp) = 15 mL
- 1 teaspoon (tsp) = 5 mL
- 1 fluid ounce (fl oz) = 30 mL
- 1 pint (pt) = 473 mL
- 1 quart (qt) = 946 mL
- 1 gallon (gal) = 3.785 L

Dry Measurements:

Cups to Grams (for common smoothie ingredients):

- 1 cup of sliced bananas = 150 g
- 1 cup of berries = 140 g
- 1 cup of spinach leaves = 30 g
- 1 cup of Greek yogurt = 245 g

Tablespoons to Grams:

- 1 tablespoon of honey = 21 g
- 1 tablespoon of peanut butter = 16 g
- 1 tablespoon of chia seeds = 10 g

Temperature (for any baked add-ins or toppings):

Fahrenheit to Celsius:

- 350°F = 177°C
- 375°F = 190°C
- 400°F = 204°C
- 425°F = 218°C

Weight:

Pounds to Kilograms:

- 1 pound (lb) = 0.4536 kilograms (kg)
- 1/2 pound = 0.2268 kg

Small Unit Conversions:

Teaspoons to Milliliters:

- 1 teaspoon = 5 mL
- 1/2 teaspoon = 2.5 mL
- 1/4 teaspoon = 1.25 mL

Note: These conversions are approximate. The weight of dry ingredients can vary depending on the ingredient's density and how it's packed.

Smoothie Shopping List

Creating delicious and nutritious smoothies starts with having the right ingredients on hand. Here's a comprehensive shopping list to help you stock up on essentials for a variety of smoothie creations:

Fruits (Fresh or Frozen):
- Bananas
- Mixed Berries (blueberries, strawberries, raspberries, blackberries)
- Mangoes
- Pineapples
- Apples
- Oranges
- Kiwis
- Avocados
- Peaches
- Pears

Vegetables:
- Spinach
- Kale
- Cucumber
- Carrots
- Beets (for adventurous palates)

Liquids:
- Almond milk (unsweetened)
- Coconut water
- Soy milk
- Dairy milk
- Fruit juices (100% juice, no added sugar)

Proteins:
- Greek yogurt (plain or flavored)
- Protein powder (whey or plant-based)
- Natural peanut or almond butter

Sweeteners (Optional):
- Honey
- Agave syrup
- Maple syrup
- Stevia

Superfoods and Supplements:
- Chia seeds
- Flaxseeds
- Hemp seeds
- Matcha powder
- Acai powder
- Spirulina
- Cocoa powder

Nuts and Seeds (Optional):
- Almonds
- Walnuts
- Pumpkin seeds
- Sunflower seeds

Spices and Extras:
- Cinnamon
- Nutmeg
- Vanilla extract
- Coconut shavings
- Granola

Frozen Items:
- Frozen fruit medley packs
- Frozen spinach or kale

Remember, you don't need to purchase every item on this list. Start with a selection of your favorite fruits, a couple of liquid options, a protein source, and maybe one or two superfoods. As you experiment with different smoothie recipes, you can gradually expand your ingredient list to include more variety. Enjoy your smoothie making!

CHAPTER 2

Detox Smoothie

🕐 **Preparation Time:** 05m

Watermelon Flush Smoothie

Ingredients

- Watermelon: 2 cups, cubed (about 300g)
- Fresh mint leaves: 1/4 cup (about 15g)
- Lime: juice of 1 medium (about 30g)
- Ice cubes: a handful (optional)

Directions

- Cube the watermelon, ensuring it is seedless. Rinse the mint leaves. Juice the lime.
- In a blender, combine the watermelon cubes, mint leaves, and lime juice. Add ice cubes if you want a colder drink.
- Blend on a medium speed for about 30-60 seconds until smooth and well-mixed.
- If the smoothie is too thick, add a small amount of water. For extra sweetness, a teaspoon of honey can be added.
- Pour into glasses and enjoy this wonderfully refreshing smoothie!

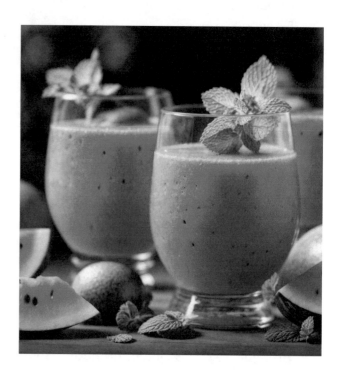

Nutritional Info

- Calories: 80 kcal
- Protein: 2 g
- Carbohydrates: 20 g
- Dietary Fiber: 1 g
- Sugars: 16 g
- Fat: 0.5 g
- Cholesterol: 0 mg
- Sodium: 3 mg
- Potassium: 270 mg
- Vitamin C: 25 mg
- Calcium: 20 mg
- Iron: 0.6 mg

Tips and Techniques

- If mint is not available, basil can provide a unique and delightful flavor. For an additional flavor twist, add a slice of ginger or a few cucumber slices.
- To add a boost of protein, include a scoop of unflavored or vanilla protein powder.
- This smoothie is best enjoyed immediately due to the watermelon's high water content. However, if needed, it can be stored in the fridge for a few hours.

Green Detox Smoothie

Ingredients

- Spinach: 2 cups (30g)
- Kale: 1 cup, stems removed (67g)
- Green apple: 1 medium, cored and chopped (182g)
- Cucumber: ½ medium, sliced (150g)
- Lemon: juice of 1 medium (44g)
- Ginger: 1-inch piece, peeled (11g)
- Cold water or coconut water: 1 cup (240ml)
- Ice cubes: a handful (optional)

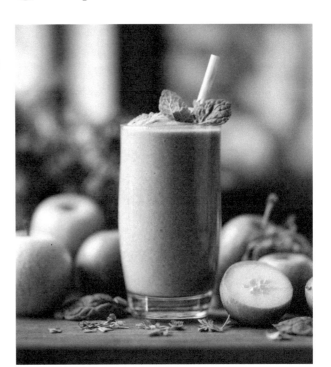

Nutritional Info

- Calories: 145 kcal
- Protein: 4 g
- Carbohydrates: 35 g
- Dietary Fiber: 6 g
- Fat: 1 g
- Saturated Fat: 0 g
- Cholesterol: 0 mg
- Sodium: 70 mg
- Potassium: 856 mg
- Vitamin A: 10,700 IU
- Vitamin C: 145 mg
- Calcium: 150 mg
- Iron: 3 mg

Directions

- Wash and Prepare Ingredients: Rinse the spinach, kale, green apple, cucumber, and lemon thoroughly. Core and chop the apple. Slice the cucumber. Juice the lemon. Peel and slice the ginger.
- Blending: In a high-speed blender, add the spinach, kale, green apple, cucumber, lemon juice, ginger, and cold water or coconut water. If you like your smoothie cold, add a handful of ice cubes.
- Blending Speed and Time: Start blending at a low speed to combine the ingredients, then gradually increase to high speed. Blend for about 60 seconds or until the smoothie is smooth and creamy.
- Taste and Adjust: Taste the smoothie. If it's too thick, add more water or coconut water. If you prefer it sweeter, you can add a teaspoon of honey or agave syrup.
- Serve Immediately: Pour the smoothie into a glass and enjoy!

Tips and Techniques

- Ingredient Alternatives: If kale is not available, you can use additional spinach or try other greens like Swiss chard. If you're not a fan of green apples, try using a ripe pear.
- Texture Adjustment: For a thinner smoothie, add more liquid. For a thicker smoothie, add more greens or apples.
- Nutrition Boost: To increase the protein content, add a scoop of your favorite protein powder or a tablespoon of chia seeds.
- Storage: This smoothie is best enjoyed fresh, but you can store it in the fridge for up to 24 hours. Just give it a good shake before drinking.

Berry Bliss Detox Smoothie

Ingredients

- Blueberries: ½ cup (74g)
- Raspberries: ½ cup (62g)
- Strawberries: ½ cup, hulled (72g)
- Acai berry puree: 2 tablespoons (30g)
- Banana: 1 small, sliced (90g)
- Almond milk or water: 1 cup (240ml)
- Ice cubes: a handful (optional)

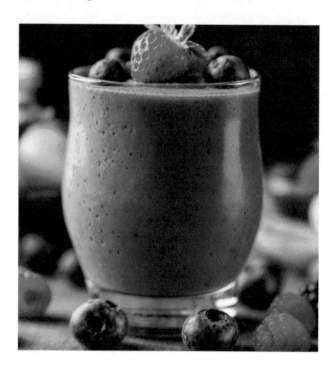

Nutritional Info

- Calories: 190 kcal
- Protein: 3 g
- Carbohydrates: 44 g
- Dietary Fiber: 9 g
- Fat: 2 g
- Saturated Fat: 0 g
- Cholesterol: 0 mg
- Sodium: 60 mg
- Potassium: 450 mg
- Vitamin C: 60 mg
- Calcium: 200 mg
- Iron: 1.5 mg

Directions

- Wash and Prepare Ingredients: Rinse the blueberries, raspberries, and strawberries. Hull the strawberries and chop them. Peel and slice the banana.
- Blending: In a blender, combine the blueberries, raspberries, strawberries, acai berry puree, banana, and almond milk or water. If you like your smoothie cold, add a handful of ice cubes.
- Blending Speed and Time: Start blending on a low speed, then increase to high. Blend for about 60 seconds or until the smoothie is smooth.
- Taste and Adjust: If the smoothie is too thick, add more almond milk or water. For extra sweetness, you can add a teaspoon of honey or maple syrup.
- Serve Immediately: Pour the smoothie into a glass and enjoy!

Tips and Techniques

- Ingredient Alternatives: If acai berry puree is not available, you can substitute with acai berry powder or extra blueberries. You can also use any plant-based milk like soy or oat milk instead of almond milk.
- Nutrition Boost: To add more protein and healthy fats, include a tablespoon of almond butter or a scoop of protein powder.
- Storage: It's best to consume this smoothie fresh, but if needed, you can store it in the refrigerator for up to 24 hours.
- Enjoy your Berry Bliss Detox Smoothie, a perfect blend of berries and banana for a healthy, delicious treat!

Tropical Turmeric Cleanser Smoothie

Ingredients

- Pineapple: 1 cup, chopped (165g)
- Mango: 1 cup, chopped (165g)
- Coconut water: 1 cup (240ml)
- Turmeric: ½ teaspoon, ground (1g)
- Fresh ginger: ½ inch piece, peeled (3g)
- Ice cubes: a handful (optional)
- Black pepper: a pinch (to enhance turmeric absorption)

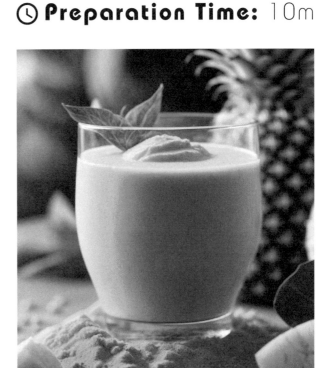

Nutritional Info

- Calories: 160 kcal
- Protein: 2 g
- Carbohydrates: 39 g
- Dietary Fiber: 4 g
- Fat: 1 g
- Saturated Fat: 0 g
- Cholesterol: 0 mg
- Sodium: 252 mg
- Potassium: 600 mg
- Vitamin C: 125 mg
- Calcium: 58 mg
- Iron: 1 mg

Directions

- Wash and Prepare Ingredients: Peel and chop the pineapple and mango. Peel the ginger.
- Blending: In a blender, add the chopped pineapple, mango, coconut water, ground turmeric, peeled ginger, and a pinch of black pepper. If you prefer a colder smoothie, add a handful of ice cubes.
- Blending Speed and Time: Blend on a low speed to start, then increase to high speed. Blend for about 60 seconds or until smooth.
- Taste and Adjust: If the smoothie is too thick, add more coconut water. For added sweetness, a teaspoon of honey can be included.
- Serve Immediately: Pour the smoothie into glasses and enjoy this tropical, health-boosting drink!

Tips and Techniques

- Ingredient Alternatives: If fresh mango or pineapple isn't available, you can use frozen fruit. You can also substitute coconut water with almond milk or regular water for a different taste.
- Nutrition Boost: For added nutritional value, include a tablespoon of chia seeds or flaxseeds.
- Storage: This smoothie is best enjoyed fresh. However, if necessary, it can be stored in the fridge for up to 24 hours. Stir or shake well before consuming.
- Relish this Tropical Turmeric Cleanser Smoothie for a delicious way to detox and nourish your body!

Beetroot & Berry Liver Cleanse Smoothie

Ingredients

- Beetroot: 1 medium, peeled and chopped (approx. 135g)
- Mixed berries (blueberries, raspberries, strawberries): 1 cup, fresh or frozen (140g)
- Lemon: juice of 1 medium (approx. 44g)
- Ginger: 1-inch piece, peeled (approx. 11g)
- Water or coconut water: 1 cup (240ml)
- Ice cubes: a handful (optional)

Nutritional Info

- Calories: 120 kcal
- Protein: 3 g
- Carbohydrates: 29 g
- Dietary Fiber: 7 g
- Fat: 0.5 g
- Saturated Fat: 0 g
- Cholesterol: 0 mg
- Sodium: 106 mg
- Potassium: 600 mg
- Vitamin C: 40 mg
- Calcium: 40 mg
- Iron: 1.5 mg

⏱ Preparation Time: 10m

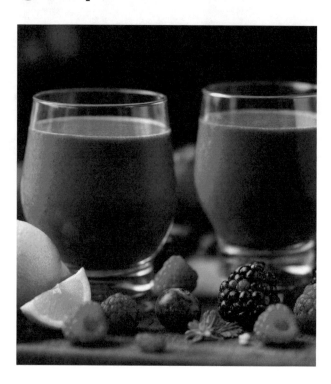

Directions

- Preparation Time: 10-15 minutes
- Prepare the Ingredients: Peel and chop the beetroot. If using fresh berries, wash them thoroughly. Juice the lemon. Peel and slice the ginger.
- Blending: In a blender, add the chopped beetroot, mixed berries, lemon juice, ginger, and water or coconut water. If you like a colder smoothie, include a handful of ice cubes.
- Blending Speed and Time: Start blending at a lower speed, then increase to high. Blend for about 60-90 seconds, until the smoothie is smooth and creamy.
- Taste and Adjust: If the smoothie is too thick, add more water or coconut water. For additional sweetness, you can add a teaspoon of honey or maple syrup.
- Serve Immediately: Pour the smoothie into a glass and enjoy your liver detox drink!

Tips and Techniques

- Ingredient Alternatives: If beetroot is not available, you can use cooked beets. Instead of mixed berries, any single type of berry can be used.
- Nutrition Boost: Add a tablespoon of ground flaxseed or a scoop of protein powder for extra nutrition.
- Storage: Best consumed fresh. If necessary, store in the fridge for up to 24 hours, but the color and texture may change slightly.
- Enjoy this nutritious Beetroot and Berry Liver Cleanse Smoothie as a part of your detox routine!

Carrot Ginger Zinger Smoothie

Ingredients

- Carrots: 2 medium, peeled and chopped (about 120g)
- Orange: 1 large, peeled and segmented (about 140g)
- Lemon: juice of 1 medium (about 44g)
- Ginger: 1-inch piece, peeled (about 11g)
- Water or orange juice: 1 cup (240ml)
- Ice cubes: a handful (optional)

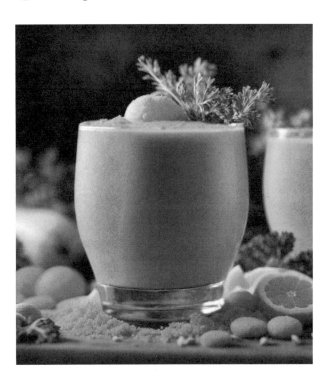

Nutritional Info

- Calories: 130 kcal
- Protein: 3 g
- Carbohydrates: 31 g
- Dietary Fiber: 7 g
- Fat: 0.5 g
- Saturated Fat: 0 g
- Sodium: 70 mg
- Potassium: 640 mg
- Vitamin A: 21000 IU
- Vitamin C: 95 mg
- Calcium: 72 mg
- Iron: 0.5 mg

Directions

- Prepare the Ingredients: Wash, peel, and chop the carrots. Peel the orange and segment it. Juice the lemon. Peel and slice the ginger.
- Blending: In a blender, add the carrots, orange segments, lemon juice, ginger, and water or orange juice. If you prefer a colder smoothie, add a handful of ice cubes.
- Blending Speed and Time: Start at a low speed, then increase to high. Blend for about 60-90 seconds until the mixture is smooth.
- Taste and Adjust: If the smoothie is too thick, add more water or orange juice. If you want more sweetness, add a teaspoon of honey.
- Serve Immediately: Pour into glasses and enjoy your fresh and zingy smoothie!

Tips and Techniques

- Ingredient Alternatives: If oranges are not available, you can substitute with clementines or mandarins. Apple juice can be used instead of orange juice for a different flavor profile.
- Nutrition Boost: For additional nutrition, add a tablespoon of chia seeds or flaxseeds.
- Storage: It's best to consume this smoothie immediately, but it can be stored in the refrigerator for up to 24 hours.
- The Carrot Ginger Zinger Smoothie is a perfect blend of flavor and nutrition, making it an excellent choice for a morning or midday boost!

Cool Cucumber Mint Smoothie

Ingredients

🕐 **Preparation Time:** 10m

- Cucumber: 1 large, chopped (about 300g)
- Fresh mint leaves: 1/4 cup (about 15g)
- Lime: juice of 1 medium (about 30g)
- Green apple: 1 medium, cored and chopped (about 180g)
- Water or coconut water: 1 cup (240ml)
- Ice cubes: a handful (optional)

Nutritional Info

- Calories: 110 kcal
- Protein: 2 g
- Carbohydrates: 27 g
- Dietary Fiber: 5 g
- Fat: 0.5 g
- Saturated Fat: 0 g
- Cholesterol: 0 mg
- Sodium: 12 mg
- Potassium: 500 mg
- Vitamin C: 22 mg
- Calcium: 48 mg
- Iron: 0.7 mg

Directions

- Prepare the Ingredients: Wash and chop the cucumber. Rinse the mint leaves. Juice the lime. Core and chop the green apple.
- Blending: In a blender, combine the cucumber, mint leaves, lime juice, green apple, and water or coconut water. Add ice cubes for a colder smoothie.
- Blending Speed and Time: Start blending at a low speed and gradually increase to high. Blend for about 60 seconds or until smooth.
- Taste and Adjust: If the smoothie is too thick, add more water or coconut water. For extra sweetness, consider adding a teaspoon of honey or agave syrup.
- Serve Immediately: Pour the smoothie into glasses and enjoy immediately for the best taste and texture!

Tips and Techniques

- Ingredient Alternatives: If green apples aren't available, you can use another variety of apple or even a pear for a similar texture and sweetness.
- Nutrition Boost: To increase the protein content, add a scoop of your favorite protein powder or a tablespoon of chia seeds.
- Storage: This smoothie is best enjoyed fresh due to the ingredients' tendency to oxidize and change flavor over time. However, you can store it in the fridge for up to 24 hours if necessary.
- The Cool Cucumber Mint Smoothie is a wonderfully light and hydrating option, perfect for a nutritious and refreshing drink!

Spicy Lemonade Smoothie

Ingredients

- Lemon: juice of 2 large lemons (about 88g)
- Cayenne pepper: 1/8 teaspoon (0.3g)
- Agave nectar: 2 tablespoons (30ml)
- Water: 2 cups (480ml)
- Ice cubes: a handful (optional)

Nutritional Info

- Calories: 50 kcal
- Protein: 0 g
- Carbohydrates: 14 g
- Dietary Fiber: 0.4 g
- Fats: 0 g
- Saturated Fat: 0 g
- Cholesterol: 0 mg
- Sodium: 2 mg
- Potassium: 75 mg
- Vitamin C: 47 mg
- Calcium: 7 mg
- Iron: 0.1 mg

⏱ Preparation Time: 05m

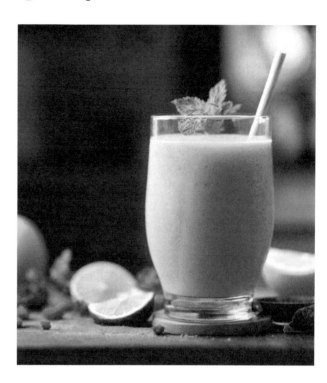

Directions

- Prepare the Ingredients: Juice the lemons. Measure the cayenne pepper and agave nectar.
- Mixing: In a blender, combine the lemon juice, cayenne pepper, agave nectar, and water. Add ice cubes if you prefer a chilled drink.
- Blending Speed and Time: Blend on a medium speed for about 30 seconds or until everything is well mixed and the drink is slightly frothy.
- Taste and Adjust: Adjust the sweetness by adding more agave nectar if desired. If it's too spicy, add more water.
- Serve Immediately: Pour into glasses and enjoy this invigorating and detoxifying smoothie!

Tips and Techniques

- Ingredient Alternatives: If agave nectar is not available, you can substitute it with honey or maple syrup. However, these alternatives might slightly change the flavor profile.
- Spice Adjustment: Be cautious with cayenne pepper as it is quite spicy. Start with a small amount and adjust according to your taste.
- Nutrition Boost: For added nutritional benefits, you can include a teaspoon of apple cider vinegar or a pinch of turmeric.
- Storage: This drink is best consumed immediately. If you need to store it, keep it in the fridge for up to 24 hours. Enjoy your Spicy Lemonade Smoothie for a refreshing and detoxifying experience!

Avocado Dream Smoothie

Ingredients

- Avocado: 1 medium, pitted and scooped (about 150g)
- Spinach: 1 cup (30g)
- Cucumber: ½ medium, chopped (about 150g)
- Coconut water: 1 cup (240ml)
- Ice cubes: a handful (optional)

Nutritional Info

- Calories: 250 kcal
- Protein: 4 g
- Carbohydrates: 20 g
- Dietary Fiber: 10 g
- Fat: 18 g
- Saturated Fat: 3 g
- Sodium: 120 mg
- Potassium: 890 mg
- Vitamin A: 2900 IU
- Vitamin C: 30 mg
- Calcium: 60 mg
- Iron: 1.5 mg

⏱ Preparation Time: 10m

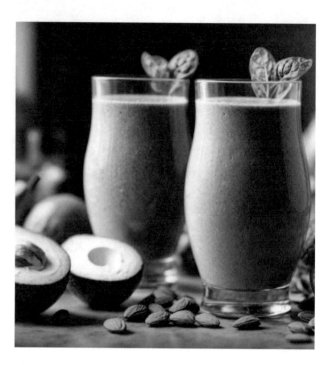

Directions

- Prepare the Ingredients: Wash the spinach and cucumber. Chop the cucumber. Cut the avocado in half, remove the pit, and scoop out the flesh.
- Blending: In a blender, combine the avocado, spinach, cucumber, and coconut water. Add ice cubes if you prefer a colder smoothie.
- Blending Speed and Time: Start blending at a low speed and increase to high. Blend for about 60 seconds until smooth and creamy.
- Taste and Adjust: If the smoothie is too thick, add more coconut water. For added sweetness, consider a teaspoon of honey or agave syrup.
- Serve Immediately: Pour the smoothie into glasses and enjoy this creamy and nutritious drink!

Tips and Techniques

- Ingredient Alternatives: If coconut water is not available, you can use almond milk or regular water. You can also add a banana for extra creaminess and sweetness.
- Nutrition Boost: To increase the protein content, add a scoop of your favorite protein powder or a tablespoon of chia seeds.
- Storage: This smoothie is best consumed immediately, but it can be stored in the refrigerator for up to 24 hours. The avocado may cause the smoothie to change color slightly.
- Savor the rich and creamy goodness of this Avocado Dream Smoothie, a perfect blend for a healthy treat!

Chia Seed Berry Yogurt Smoothie

Ingredients

- Mixed berries (blueberries, raspberries, strawberries): 1 cup, fresh or frozen (140g)
- Greek yogurt: 1 cup (245g)
- Chia seeds: 2 tablespoons (24g)
- Honey: 1 tablespoon (15ml)
- Water or almond milk: 1/2 cup (120ml)
- Ice cubes: a handful (optional)

⏱ Preparation Time: 10m

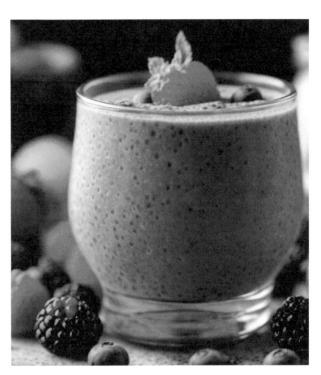

Nutritional Info

- Calories: 290 kcal
- Protein: 20 g
- Carbohydrates: 38 g
- Dietary Fiber: 8 g
- Sugars: 24 g
- Fat: 8 g
- Saturated Fat: 1 g
- Cholesterol: 10 mg
- Sodium: 60 mg
- Potassium: 360 mg
- Vitamin C: 30 mg
- Calcium: 250 mg
- Iron: 2 mg

Directions

- Prepare the Ingredients: If using fresh berries, wash them thoroughly. Measure the Greek yogurt, chia seeds, and honey.
- Soaking Chia Seeds: (Optional) For a smoother texture, soak chia seeds in water or almond milk for about 10 minutes until they become gel-like.
- Blending: In a blender, combine the mixed berries, Greek yogurt, soaked chia seeds, honey, and water or almond milk. Add ice cubes for a colder smoothie.
- Blending Speed and Time: Blend on a medium to high speed for about 60 seconds, until the mixture is smooth and creamy.
- Taste and Adjust: If the smoothie is too thick, add more water or almond milk. Adjust sweetness with additional honey if desired.
- Serve Immediately: Pour the smoothie into glasses and enjoy your protein-rich, detoxifying treat!

Tips and Techniques

- Ingredient Alternatives: If Greek yogurt is not available, any plain or vanilla yogurt can be used. You can also use any plant-based milk instead of almond milk.
- Nutrition Boost: Add a tablespoon of ground flaxseed or a scoop of protein powder for extra nutrition.
- Storage: Best consumed fresh. However, if necessary, store in the refrigerator for up to 24 hours.
- Relish this Chia Seed Berry Yogurt Smoothie, a perfect combination of taste and health benefits!

Pomegranate Beet Smoothie

Ingredients

- Pomegranate juice: 1 cup (240ml)
- Cooked beet: 1 medium, peeled and chopped (about 135g)
- Orange: 1 large, peeled and segmented (about 140g)
- Ginger: 1-inch piece, peeled (about 11g)
- Ice cubes: a handful (optional)

⏱ Preparation Time: 10m

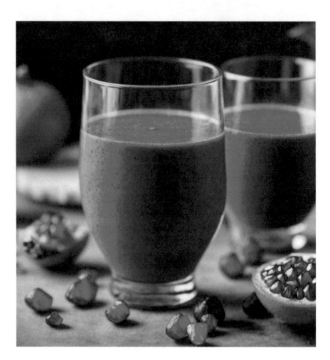

Nutritional Info

- Calories: 180 kcal
- Protein: 3 g
- Carbohydrates: 42 g
- Dietary Fiber: 7 g
- Fat: 0.5 g
- Saturated Fat: 0 g
- Cholesterol: 0 mg
- Sodium: 85 mg
- Potassium: 660 mg
- Vitamin C: 70 mg
- Calcium: 40 mg
- Iron: 1.2 mg

Directions

- Prepare the Ingredients: If using a fresh beet, cook it until tender, peel, and chop. Peel and segment the orange. Peel and slice the ginger.
- Blending: In a blender, combine the pomegranate juice, cooked beet, orange segments, and ginger. Add ice cubes for a chilled smoothie.
- Blending Speed and Time: Blend on medium to high speed for about 60-90 seconds until the mixture is smooth.
- Taste and Adjust: If the smoothie is too thick, add more pomegranate juice or water. Adjust sweetness if necessary with a little honey or agave syrup.
- Serve Immediately: Pour the smoothie into glasses and enjoy this antioxidant-rich drink!

Tips and Techniques

- Ingredient Alternatives: If pomegranate juice is not available, you can use cranberry juice or a blend of red fruit juices. For a sweeter smoothie, add an apple or a banana.
- Nutrition Boost: For additional fiber and omega-3 fatty acids, add a tablespoon of ground flaxseed or chia seeds.
- Storage: This smoothie is best enjoyed fresh, but it can be stored in the refrigerator for up to 24 hours. Note that the color and texture may change slightly due to the ingredients.
- Savor the delightful and nutritious blend of this Pomegranate Beet Smoothie, a perfect drink for detox and health!

Almond Butter & Banana Smoothie

Ingredients

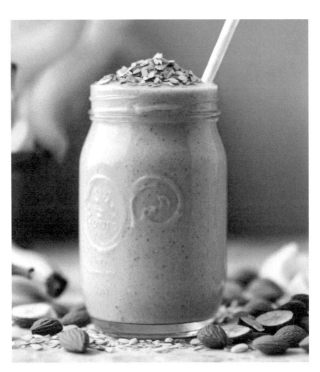

⏱ Preparation Time: 10m

- Banana: 1 large, ripe (about 120g)
- Almond butter: 2 tablespoons (32g)
- Almond milk: 1 cup (240ml)
- Ground flax seeds: 1 tablespoon (7g)
- Ice cubes: a handful (optional)

Nutritional Info

- Calories: 330 kcal
- Protein: 9 g
- Carbohydrates: 37 g
- Dietary Fiber: 7 g
- Sugars: 18 g
- Fat: 18 g
- Saturated Fat: 1.5 g
- Cholesterol: 0 mg
- Sodium: 180 mg
- Potassium: 600 mg
- Vitamin C: 10 mg
- Calcium: 300 mg
- Iron: 1.8 mg

Directions

- Prepare the Ingredients: Peel the banana. Measure the almond butter and ground flax seeds.
- Blending: In a blender, add the banana, almond butter, almond milk, and ground flax seeds. Include ice cubes for a chilled smoothie.
- Blending Speed and Time: Blend at a high speed for about 60 seconds until the mixture becomes smooth and creamy.
- Taste and Adjust: If the smoothie is too thick, add more almond milk. For additional sweetness, consider adding a teaspoon of honey or maple syrup.
- Serve Immediately: Pour the smoothie into a glass and enjoy this nourishing and delicious drink!

Tips and Techniques

- Ingredient Alternatives: If almond butter is not available, you can use peanut butter or cashew butter. Similarly, any plant-based milk like soy or oat milk can replace almond milk.
- Nutrition Boost: For extra protein, add a scoop of your favorite protein powder. You can also add a handful of spinach or kale for added nutrients without significantly altering the flavor.
- Storage: This smoothie is best consumed immediately. If needed, it can be stored in the refrigerator for up to 24 hours, but it's best to give it a good stir or shake before consuming.
- The Almond Butter & Banana Detox Smoothie is not only delicious but also packed with healthy fats and fibers, making it an excellent choice for a fulfilling and healthy treat!

CHAPTER 3

Smoothies for Weight Loss

🕐 **Preparation Time:** 10m

Berry Oat Breakfast Smoothie

Ingredients

- Mixed berries: 140g
- Rolled oats: 1/3 cup (30g)
- Greek yogurt: 1/2 cup (120g)
- Almond milk: 1 cup (240ml)
- Ice cubes: a handful (optional)

Directions

- If using fresh berries, wash them thoroughly. Measure the rolled oats, Greek yogurt, and almond milk.
- In a blender, add the mixed berries, rolled oats, Greek yogurt, and almond milk. Include ice cubes if you prefer a chilled smoothie.
- Blend on a high speed for about 60 seconds until all ingredients are well combined and the mixture is smooth. If the smoothie is too thick, add more almond milk. For added sweetness, consider a teaspoon of honey or maple syrup.
- Pour into a glass and enjoy your nutritious and satisfying breakfast smoothie!

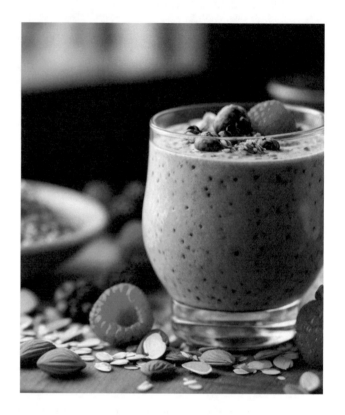

Nutritional Info

- Calories: 290 kcal
- Protein: 15 g
- Carbohydrates: 50 g
- Dietary Fiber: 7 g
- Sugars: 20 g
- Fat: 4 g
- Saturated Fat: 0.5 g
- Cholesterol: 5 mg
- Sodium: 125 mg
- Potassium: 400 mg
- Vitamin A: 100 IU
- Vitamin C: 30 mg
- Calcium: 300 mg
- Iron: 2 mg

Tips and Techniques

- If almond milk is not available, you can use any other plant-based milk, such as soy or oat milk. If Greek yogurt is not an option, any plain yogurt will work.
- To increase the protein content or add healthy fats, add a tablespoon of chia seeds, hemp seeds, or a scoop of protein powder.
- This smoothie can be stored in the refrigerator for up to 24 hours, making it a convenient breakfast option. Shake well before drinking if stored.

Green Tea & Berry Metabolism Booster

Ingredients

- Brewed green tea, cooled: 1 cup (240ml)
- Mixed berries (strawberries, blueberries, raspberries): 1 cup, fresh or frozen (140g)
- Honey: 1 tablespoon (15ml)
- Ice cubes: a handful (optional)

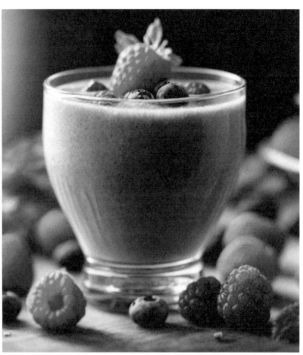

Nutritional Info

- Calories: 90 kcal
- Protein: 1 g
- Carbohydrates: 22 g
- Dietary Fiber: 3 g
- Sugars: 17 g
- Fat: 0.5 g
- Saturated Fat: 0 g
- Cholesterol: 0 mg
- Sodium: 7 mg
- Potassium: 120 mg
- Vitamin C: 35 mg
- Calcium: 20 mg
- Iron: 0.5 mg

Directions

- Prepare the Ingredients: Brew a cup of green tea and allow it to cool. Wash the mixed berries if they are fresh.
- Blending: In a blender, combine the cooled green tea, mixed berries, and honey. Add ice cubes if you want a colder smoothie.
- Blending Speed and Time: Blend on a medium to high speed for about 60 seconds until smooth.
- Taste and Adjust: Adjust the sweetness by adding more honey if needed.
- Serve Immediately: Pour into a glass and enjoy your metabolism-boosting smoothie!

Tips and Techniques

- Ingredient Alternatives: If honey is not available, you can use agave syrup or a few drops of stevia for a low-calorie option.
- Nutrition Boost: Add a scoop of protein powder or a tablespoon of chia seeds for extra nutrition.
- Storage: Best consumed immediately. However, if needed, it can be stored in the refrigerator for a few hours.
- This Green Tea and Berry Metabolism Booster Smoothie is not only delicious but also a great way to help boost your metabolism naturally!

Spinach & Avocado Power Smoothie

Ingredients

- Spinach: 1 cup (30g)
- Avocado: 1/2 medium, pitted and scooped (about 75g)
- Banana: 1 medium, ripe (about 120g)
- Almond milk: 1 cup (240ml)
- Ice cubes: a handful (optional)

Nutritional Info

- Calories: 250 kcal
- Protein: 5 g
- Carbohydrates: 32 g
- Dietary Fiber: 9 g
- Sugars: 13 g
- Fat: 14 g
- Saturated Fat: 2 g

- Cholesterol: 0 mg
- Sodium: 180 mg
- Potassium: 890 mg
- Vitamin A: 4700 IU
- Vitamin C: 20 mg
- Calcium: 300 mg
- Iron: 2 mg

⏱ Preparation Time: 10m

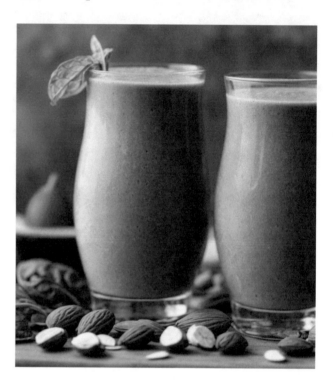

Directions

- Prepare the Ingredients: Wash the spinach leaves. Cut the avocado in half, remove the pit, and scoop out the flesh. Peel the banana.
- Blending: In a blender, add the spinach, avocado, banana, and almond milk. Include ice cubes if you prefer a colder smoothie.
- Blending Speed and Time: Blend on a high speed for about 60 seconds or until the mixture becomes smooth and creamy.
- Taste and Adjust: If the smoothie is too thick, add more almond milk to reach your desired consistency.
- Serve Immediately: Pour the smoothie into a glass and enjoy this energizing and nutritious drink!

Tips and Techniques

- Ingredient Alternatives: If almond milk is not available, you can use any other plant-based milk, such as soy or oat milk. You can also add a scoop of protein powder or a tablespoon of chia seeds for added protein and omega-3 fatty acids.
- Nutrition Boost: For extra fiber and nutrients, you can add a small handful of kale or a tablespoon of flaxseeds.
- Storage: This smoothie is best consumed immediately, but it can be stored in the refrigerator for up to 24 hours. Stir well before drinking if stored.
- The Spinach and Avocado Power Smoothie is a wonderfully creamy and satisfying drink, perfect for a healthy start to your day or as a nutrient-packed snack!

Kale & Pineapple Slim-Down Smoothie

Ingredients

- Kale: 1 cup, stems removed (67g)
- Pineapple: 1 cup, chopped (165g)
- Banana: 1 medium, ripe (120g)
- Greek yogurt: 1/2 cup (120g)
- Ice cubes: a handful (optional)

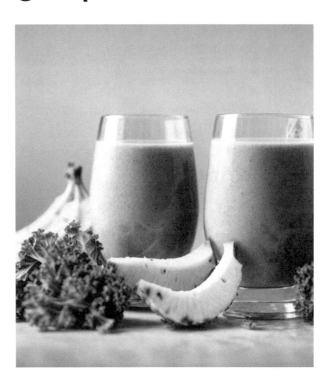

Nutritional Info

- Calories: 210 kcal
- Protein: 11 g
- Carbohydrates: 42 g
- Dietary Fiber: 4 g
- Sugars: 24 g
- Fat: 1 g
- Saturated Fat: 0.5 g

- Cholesterol: 5 mg
- Sodium: 70 mg
- Potassium: 700 mg
- Vitamin A: 6700 IU
- Vitamin C: 95 mg
- Calcium: 150 mg
- Iron: 1.5 mg

Directions

- Prepare the Ingredients: Rinse the kale leaves and remove the stems. Chop the pineapple and peel the banana.
- Blending: In a blender, combine the kale, pineapple, banana, and Greek yogurt. Add ice cubes if you prefer a chilled smoothie.
- Blending Speed and Time: Blend on a high speed for about 60 seconds until the mixture is smooth.
- Taste and Adjust: If the smoothie is too thick, add a little water or additional Greek yogurt to reach your desired consistency.
- Serve Immediately: Pour into a glass and enjoy this refreshing and slimming smoothie!

Tips and Techniques

- Ingredient Alternatives: If Greek yogurt is not available, you can use any plain yogurt or a plant-based yogurt alternative. For added sweetness, consider a teaspoon of honey or agave syrup.
- Nutrition Boost: Add a tablespoon of chia seeds or flaxseeds for extra fiber and omega-3 fatty acids.
- Storage: Best consumed fresh. However, if needed, it can be stored in the refrigerator for up to 24 hours. Shake or stir well before consuming.
- The Kale and Pineapple Slim-Down Smoothie is a perfect blend for those looking for a delicious, healthy drink that supports weight loss goals!

Apple & Cinnamon Detox Smoothie

Ingredients

- Green apple: 1 medium, cored and chopped (about 180g)
- Cinnamon: 1/2 teaspoon (1g)
- Spinach: 1 cup (30g)
- Almond milk, unsweetened: 1 cup (240ml)
- Ice cubes: a handful (optional)

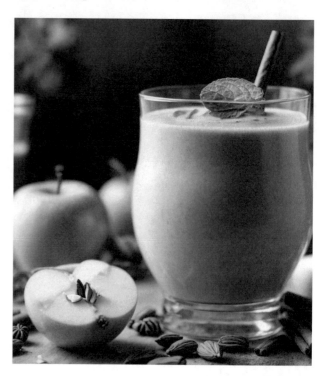

Nutritional Info

- Calories: 120 kcal
- Protein: 3 g
- Carbohydrates: 26 g
- Dietary Fiber: 5 g
- Sugars: 17 g
- Fat: 2.5 g
- Saturated Fat: 0 g

- Cholesterol: 0 mg
- Sodium: 180 mg
- Potassium: 400 mg
- Vitamin A: 2900 IU
- Vitamin C: 14 mg
- Calcium: 300 mg
- Iron: 1.5 mg

Directions

- Prepare the Ingredients: Wash and chop the green apple (leave the skin on for extra fiber). Measure the cinnamon. Wash the spinach leaves.
- Blending: In a blender, combine the chopped green apple, cinnamon, spinach, and almond milk. Add ice cubes for a colder smoothie.
- Blending Speed and Time: Blend on a high speed for about 60 seconds until the mixture is smooth.
- Taste and Adjust: If the smoothie is too thick, add more almond milk. For additional sweetness, you can add a teaspoon of honey or agave syrup, although this will increase the sugar content.
- Serve Immediately: Pour into a glass and enjoy this detoxifying and weight-loss-friendly smoothie!

Tips and Techniques

- Ingredient Alternatives: If green apple is not available, any type of apple can be used. The cinnamon can be adjusted to taste, and you can use any plant-based milk instead of almond milk.
- Nutrition Boost: Add a tablespoon of chia seeds or flaxseeds for added fiber and omega-3 fatty acids.
- Storage: Best consumed fresh. However, it can be stored in the refrigerator for up to 24 hours if necessary.
- The Apple and Cinnamon Detox Delight Smoothie is an excellent choice for those looking to support weight loss and detoxification with a delicious and healthy drink!

Citrus and Ginger Zing Smoothie

Ingredients

⏱ Preparation Time: 10m

- Oranges: 2 medium, peeled and segmented (about 280g)
- Ginger: 1-inch piece, peeled (about 11g)
- Carrot: 1 medium, peeled and chopped (about 60g)
- Protein powder: 1 scoop (varies by brand, typically around 30g)
- Water or almond milk: 1 cup (240ml)
- Ice cubes: a handful (optional)

Nutritional Info

- Calories: 220-250 kcal
- Protein: 15-25 g
  Carbohydrates: 35 g
- Dietary Fiber: 7 g
- Sugars: 22 g
- Fat: 1 g
- Saturated Fat: 0 g

- Cholesterol: 0 mg
- Sodium: 100 mg
- Potassium: 650 mg
- Vitamin A: 10500 IU
- Vitamin C: 140 mg
- Calcium: 200 mg
- Iron: 1 mg

Directions

- Prepare the Ingredients: Peel and segment the oranges. Peel and chop the carrot. Peel and slice the ginger.
- Blending: In a blender, add the orange segments, chopped carrot, ginger, protein powder, and water or almond milk. Add ice cubes for a colder smoothie.
- Blending Speed and Time: Blend on high speed for about 60-90 seconds until the mixture is smooth.
- Taste and Adjust: If the smoothie is too thick, add more water or almond milk. Adjust sweetness if necessary, but be mindful of added sugars.
- Serve Immediately: Pour into a glass and enjoy this nutritious and metabolism-boosting smoothie!

Tips and Techniques

- Ingredient Alternatives: If oranges are not available, you can use tangerines, clementines, or grapefruit. Any type of protein powder (whey, pea, hemp, etc.) can be used based on dietary preferences.
- Nutrition Boost: Add a handful of spinach or kale for added vitamins and minerals without significantly altering the taste.
- Storage: This smoothie is best enjoyed fresh. If necessary, it can be stored in the refrigerator for a few hours, but it's best to drink it as soon as possible after blending.
- The Citrus and Ginger Zing Smoothie is a fantastic choice for those looking for a delicious, high-protein, and weight loss-friendly beverage!

Grapefruit & Raspberry Fat Fighter

Ingredients

- Grapefruit: 1 medium, peeled and segmented (about 230g)
- Raspberries: 1 cup, fresh or frozen (123g)
- Greek yogurt, low-fat or non-fat: 1/2 cup (120g)
- Honey: 1 teaspoon (7ml)
- Ice cubes: a handful (optional)

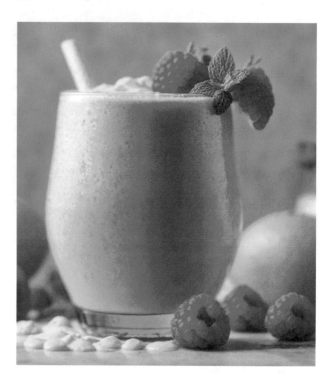

Nutritional Info

- Calories: 200 kcal
- Protein: 10 g
- Carbohydrates: 40 g
- Dietary Fiber: 6 g
- Sugars: 30 g
- Fat: 1 g
- Saturated Fat: 0.5 g
- Cholesterol: 5 mg
- Sodium: 60 mg
- Potassium: 500 mg
- Vitamin A: 3000 IU
- Vitamin C: 100 mg
- Calcium: 150 mg
- Iron: 1 mg

Directions

- Prepare the Ingredients: Peel and segment the grapefruit, removing as much of the white pith as possible to reduce bitterness. If using fresh raspberries, wash them thoroughly.
- Blending: In a blender, combine the grapefruit segments, raspberries, Greek yogurt, and honey. Add ice cubes if you prefer a chilled smoothie.
- Blending Speed and Time: Blend on high speed for about 60 seconds, or until the mixture is smooth.
- Taste and Adjust: If the smoothie is too tart, add a bit more honey. If it's too thick, add a little water or more Greek yogurt.
- Serve Immediately: Pour into glasses and enjoy this fat-fighting, delicious smoothie!

Tips and Techniques

- Ingredient Alternatives: If grapefruit is not available or if you prefer a different citrus fruit, oranges or tangerines can be a good substitute. For a vegan option, plant-based yogurt can replace Greek yogurt.
- Nutrition Boost: Add a tablespoon of chia seeds or ground flaxseeds for additional fiber and omega-3 fatty acids.
- Storage: It's best to drink this smoothie fresh, but if needed, you can store it in the refrigerator for a few hours. Be sure to stir well before drinking, as separation may occur.
- The Grapefruit and Raspberry Fat Fighter Smoothie is a great choice for anyone looking for a tasty, nutritious, and weight-loss-friendly beverage!

Blueberry & Chia Seed Slimmer

Ingredients

- Blueberries: 1 cup, fresh or frozen (148g)
- Chia seeds: 2 tablespoons (24g)
- Banana: 1 medium, ripe (about 120g)
- Almond milk, unsweetened: 1 cup (240ml)
- Ice cubes: a handful (optional)

Nutritional Info

- Calories: 280 kcal
- Protein: 6 g
- Carbohydrates: 50 g
- Dietary Fiber: 14 g
- Sugars: 22 g
- Fat: 9 g
- Saturated Fat: 0.5 g
- Cholesterol: 0 mg
- Sodium: 180 mg
- Potassium: 450 mg
- Vitamin C: 15 mg
- Calcium: 350 mg
- Iron: 2.5 mg

⏱ Preparation Time: 10m

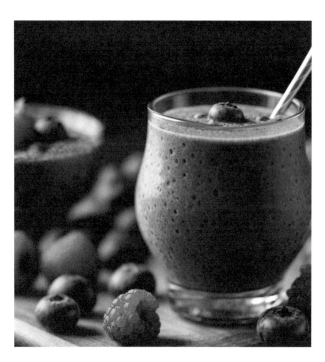

Directions

- Prepare the Ingredients: If using fresh blueberries, wash them thoroughly. Peel the banana.
- Blending: In a blender, add the blueberries, chia seeds, banana, and almond milk. Include ice cubes if you want a colder smoothie.
- Blending Speed and Time: Blend on high speed for about 60 seconds, or until the mixture is smooth and the chia seeds are well incorporated.
- Taste and Adjust: If the smoothie is too thick, add more almond milk. If additional sweetness is desired, consider adding a teaspoon of honey or agave syrup.
- Serve Immediately: Pour into glasses and enjoy this blueberry and chia seed delight!

Tips and Techniques

- Ingredient Alternatives: If almond milk is not available, any other plant-based milk like soy or oat milk can be used. Frozen blueberries are a great alternative to fresh ones and can make the smoothie colder and thicker.
- Nutrition Boost: For added protein, include a scoop of your favorite protein powder. You can also add a handful of spinach or kale for extra nutrients without significantly altering the flavor.
- Storage: This smoothie is best consumed fresh. However, if needed, it can be stored in the refrigerator for up to 24 hours. Give it a good stir or shake before consuming.
- The Blueberry and Chia Seed Slimmer Smoothie is an excellent choice for those looking for a tasty, healthy, and weight-loss-friendly beverage!

Peach & Flaxseed Digestive Aid

Ingredients

- Peaches: 2 medium, ripe and sliced (about 300g)
- Ground flaxseed: 2 tablespoons (14g)
- Greek yogurt, low-fat or non-fat: 1/2 cup (120g)
- Cinnamon: 1/4 teaspoon (0.5g)
- Ice cubes: a handful (optional)

Nutritional Info

- Calories: 220 kcal
- Protein: 12 g
- Carbohydrates: 32 g
- Dietary Fiber: 7 g
- Sugars: 22 g
- Fat: 6 g
- Saturated Fat: 0.5 g
- Cholesterol: 5 mg
- Sodium: 50 mg
- Potassium: 500 mg
- Vitamin A: 1000 IU
- Vitamin C: 10 mg
- Calcium: 150 mg
- Iron: 1.5 mg

⏱ Preparation Time: 10m

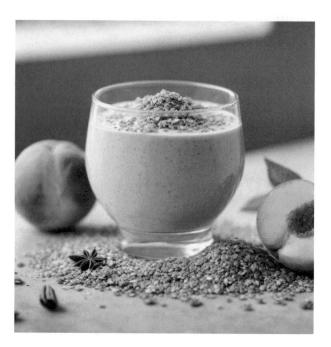

Directions

- Prepare the Ingredients: Slice the peaches (fresh or frozen can be used). Measure the ground flaxseed and cinnamon.
- Blending: In a blender, combine the peach slices, ground flaxseed, Greek yogurt, and cinnamon. Add ice cubes if you prefer a chilled smoothie.
- Blending Speed and Time: Blend on high speed for about 60 seconds, or until the mixture is smooth and creamy.
- Taste and Adjust: If the smoothie is too thick, add a little water or more Greek yogurt. For added sweetness, a teaspoon of honey or agave syrup can be included. Pour into glasses and enjoy your digestive-friendly and weight-loss-supporting smoothie!

Tips and Techniques

- Ingredient Alternatives: If peaches are not in season, you can use canned peaches (in natural juice) or another soft, ripe fruit like nectarines or apricots. If you're dairy-free, you can substitute Greek yogurt with a plant-based yogurt.
- Nutrition Boost: To enhance the protein content or add omega-3 fatty acids, consider adding a scoop of protein powder or a tablespoon of chia seeds.
- Storage: Best consumed immediately, but if necessary, it can be stored in the refrigerator for up to 24 hours. Stir well before drinking.
- The Peach and Flaxseed Digestive Aid Smoothie is a delicious, nutritious, and weight loss-friendly option, perfect for a healthy start to your day or as a satisfying snack!

Strawberry & Spinach Detox Smoothie

Ingredients

- Strawberries: 1 cup, fresh or frozen (144g)
- Spinach: 1 cup, fresh (30g)
- Greek yogurt, low-fat or non-fat: 1/2 cup (120g)
- Lemon: juice of 1 medium (about 30g)
- Ice cubes: a handful (optional)

Nutritional Info

- Calories: 140 kcal
- Protein: 10 g
- Carbohydrates: 22 g
- Dietary Fiber: 4 g
- Sugars: 13 g
- Fat: 1 g
- Saturated Fat: 0.5 g

- Cholesterol: 5 mg
- Sodium: 70 mg
- Potassium: 450 mg
- Vitamin A: 2900 IU
- Vitamin C: 95 mg
- Calcium: 150 mg
- Iron: 2 mg

⏱ Preparation Time: 10m

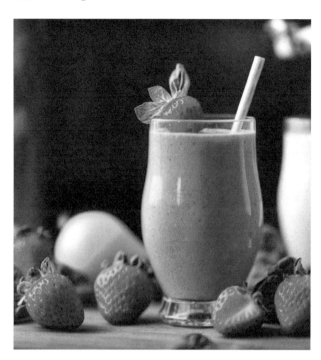

Directions

- Prepare the Ingredients: Wash the strawberries and spinach. If using fresh strawberries, remove the stems. Juice the lemon.
- Blending: In a blender, combine the strawberries, spinach, Greek yogurt, and lemon juice. Add ice cubes for a colder smoothie.
- Blending Speed and Time: Blend on high speed for about 60 seconds until the mixture is smooth.
- Taste and Adjust: If the smoothie is too thick, add a little water or more Greek yogurt. For added sweetness, consider a teaspoon of honey or agave syrup.
- Serve Immediately: Pour into glasses and enjoy this detoxifying and weight loss-friendly smoothie!

Tips and Techniques

- Ingredient Alternatives: If strawberries are not available, you can use other berries like raspberries or blueberries. Plant-based yogurt can be used instead of Greek yogurt as a vegan option.
- Nutrition Boost: Add a tablespoon of chia seeds or ground flaxseeds for extra fiber and omega-3 fatty acids.
- Storage: This smoothie is best enjoyed fresh. However, if necessary, it can be stored in the refrigerator for up to 24 hours.
- The Strawberry and Spinach Detox Smoothie is a delightful choice for anyone in the USA looking for a tasty, nutritious, and weight-loss-supportive beverage!

Celery & Apple Green Smoothie

Ingredients

🕐 **Preparation Time:** 10m

- Celery: 2 stalks, chopped (about 100g)
- Green apple: 1 medium, cored and chopped (about 180g)
- Cucumber: 1/2 medium, chopped (about 150g)
- Spinach: 1 cup, fresh (30g)
- Water or coconut water: 1 cup (240ml)
- Ice cubes: a handful (optional)

Nutritional Info

- Calories: 100 kcal
- Protein: 3 g
- Carbohydrates: 23 g
- Dietary Fiber: 5 g
- Sugars: 15 g
- Fat: 0.5 g
- Saturated Fat: 0 g
- Cholesterol: 0 mg
- Sodium: 125 mg
- Potassium: 700 mg
- Vitamin A: 2900 IU
- Vitamin C: 30 mg
- Calcium: 80 mg
- Iron: 2 mg

Directions

- Prepare the Ingredients: Wash and chop the celery, green apple, and cucumber. Rinse the spinach leaves.
- Blending: In a blender, combine the chopped celery, green apple, cucumber, spinach, and water or coconut water. Add ice cubes for a chilled smoothie.
- Blending Speed and Time: Blend on high speed for about 60 seconds, or until the mixture is smooth.
- Taste and Adjust: If the smoothie is too thick, add more water or coconut water. For added sweetness, a teaspoon of honey or agave syrup can be included.
- Serve Immediately: Pour into glasses and enjoy this refreshing and weight loss-friendly green smoothie!

Tips and Techniques

- Ingredient Alternatives: If green apple is not available, you can use another variety of apples or even a pear for a similar texture and sweetness.
- Nutrition Boost: To increase the protein content, add a scoop of your favorite protein powder or a tablespoon of chia seeds.
- Storage: This smoothie is best enjoyed fresh due to the ingredients' tendency to oxidize and change flavor over time. However, it can be stored in the fridge for a few hours if necessary.
- The Celery and Apple Green Smoothie is an excellent choice for those in the USA looking for a nutritious, delicious, and weight loss-supportive beverage!

CHAPTER 4

Vegan Smoothie Delights

🕐 **Preparation Time:** 10m

Spicy Ginger Vegan Smoothie

Ingredients

- Fresh ginger: 1-inch piece, peeled and grated
- Carrot: 1 large, peeled and chopped
- Orange: 1 large, peeled and segmented
- Almond milk: 1 cup (unsweetened)
- Ice cubes: a handful (optional)

Directions

- Peel and grate the ginger. Peel and chop the carrot. Peel and segment the orange.
- In a blender, combine the grated ginger, chopped carrot, orange segments, and almond milk. Add ice cubes if you prefer a chilled smoothie.
- Blend on high speed for about 60 seconds or until the mixture is smooth and the ingredients are well combined.
- If the smoothie is too thick, add more almond milk. If you prefer more sweetness, add a small amount of agave syrup or maple syrup. Pour into glasses and enjoy a refreshing smoothie!

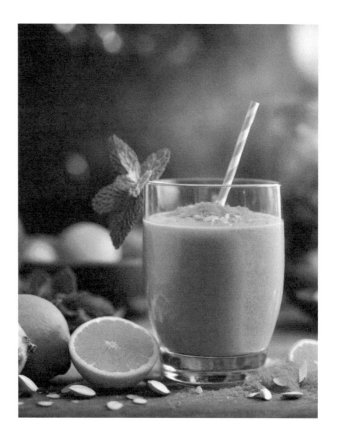

Nutritional Info

- Calories: 120 kcal
- Protein: 3 g
- Carbohydrates: 27 g
- Dietary Fiber: 6 g
- Sugars: 17 g
- Fat: 2 g
- Saturated Fat: 0 g
- Cholesterol: 0 mg
- Sodium: 180 mg
- Potassium: 600 mg
- Vitamin A: 21000 IU
- Vitamin C: 70 mg
- Calcium: 300 mg
- Iron: 0.5 mg

Tips and Techniques

- If almond milk is not available, you can use any other plant-based milk like soy or oat milk. Adding a banana can make the smoothie creamier and sweeter.
- For added nutrients, consider including a tablespoon of flaxseeds or a handful of spinach.
- This smoothie is best enjoyed fresh, but it can be stored in the refrigerator for up to 24 hours. Stir well before drinking.

Kiwi Berry Fusion Vegan Smoothie

Ingredients

- Kiwi: 2 medium, peeled and sliced
- Blueberries: 1 cup, fresh or frozen
- Spinach: 1 cup, fresh
- Rice milk: 1 cup (can be substituted with another plant-based milk if preferred)
- Ice cubes: a handful (optional, recommended if using fresh blueberries)

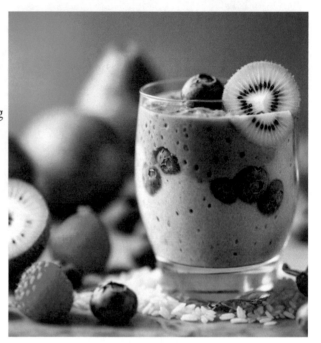

Nutritional Info

- Calories: 180 kcal
- Protein: 3 g
- Carbohydrates: 42 g
- Dietary Fiber: 5 g
- Sugars: 25 g
- Fat: 1 g
- Saturated Fat: 0 g
- Cholesterol: 0 mg
- Sodium: 70 mg
- Potassium: 500 mg
- Vitamin A: 2900 IU
- Vitamin C: 160 mg
- Calcium: 30 mg
- Iron: 1.5 mg

Directions

- Prepare the Ingredients: Peel and slice the kiwis. If using fresh blueberries, wash them thoroughly. Rinse the spinach leaves.
- Blending: In a blender, add the sliced kiwi, blueberries, spinach, and rice milk. Include ice cubes for a more refreshing and chilled smoothie.
- Blending Speed and Time: Blend on high speed for about 60 seconds, or until the mixture is smooth and well combined.
- Taste and Adjust: If the smoothie is too thick, add more rice milk. If you prefer it sweeter, consider adding a teaspoon of agave syrup or maple syrup.
- Serve Immediately: Pour into glasses and enjoy your fresh and vibrant "Kiwi Berry Fusion" smoothie!

Tips and Techniques

- Ingredient Alternatives: If rice milk is not available, you can use any other plant-based milk, such as almond or soy milk. Adding a banana can make the smoothie creamier and sweeter.
- Nutrition Boost: For added nutrients, you can include a tablespoon of chia seeds or a scoop of your favorite plant-based protein powder.
- Storage: This smoothie is best enjoyed fresh. However, if needed, you can store it in the refrigerator for up to 24 hours. Shake well before drinking if it has been stored.
- The "Kiwi Berry Fusion" vegan smoothie is a perfect blend of taste and nutrition, making it an excellent choice for a healthy, plant-based diet!

Berry Zen Blend Vegan Smoothie

Ingredients

- Blackberries: 1/3 cup, fresh or frozen
- Raspberries: 1/3 cup, fresh or frozen
- Blueberries: 1/3 cup, fresh or frozen
- Pomegranate juice: 1 cup (ensure it's pure and without added sugars for a vegan option)
- Ice cubes: a handful (optional, especially if using frozen berries)

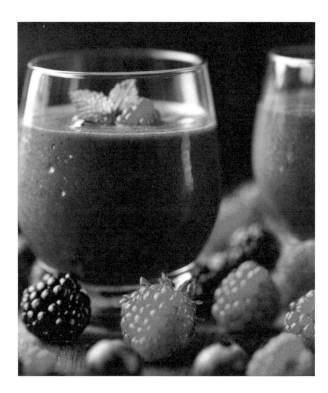

Nutritional Info

- Calories: 140 kcal
- Protein: 2 g
- Carbohydrates: 34 g
- Dietary Fiber: 8 g
- Sugars: 24 g
- Fat: 1 g
- Saturated Fat: 0 g

- Cholesterol: 0 mg
- Sodium: 15 mg
- Potassium: 300 mg
- Vitamin C: 30 mg
- Calcium: 20 mg
- Iron: 0.8 mg

Directions

- Prepare the Ingredients: If using fresh berries, wash them thoroughly.
- Blending: In a blender, add the blackberries, raspberries, blueberries, and pomegranate juice. Include ice cubes if you prefer a chilled smoothie.
- Blending Speed and Time: Blend on high speed for about 60 seconds, or until the mixture is smooth and the berries are fully blended.
- Taste and Adjust: If the smoothie is too thick, add more pomegranate juice or a little water.
- Serve Immediately: Pour into glasses and enjoy your refreshing "Berry Zen Blend" smoothie!

Tips and Techniques

- Ingredient Alternatives: If pomegranate juice is not available, you can substitute it with cranberry juice or a blend of red fruit juices.
- Nutrition Boost: For added nutrients, consider adding a tablespoon of ground flaxseed or chia seeds.
- Storage: This smoothie is best enjoyed fresh, but if needed, it can be stored in the refrigerator for up to 24 hours. Make sure to stir well before drinking.
- The "Berry Zen Blend" smoothie is a delightful way to enjoy a variety of berries in one glass, offering a wealth of health benefits and delicious flavors!

Chia Fresh Kick Vegan Smoothie

Ingredients

- Chia seeds: 2 tablespoons
- Fresh mango: 1 cup, cubed
- Kale: 1 cup, stems removed and chopped
- Coconut water: 1 cup (without added sugars)
- Ice cubes: a handful (optional)

🕐 Preparation Time: 10m

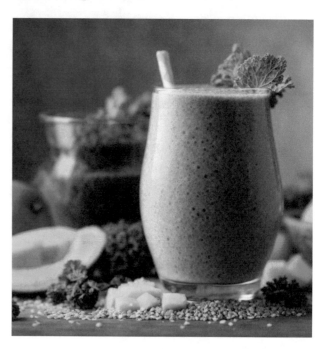

Nutritional Info

- Calories: 180 kcal
- Protein: 4 g
- Carbohydrates: 36 g
- Dietary Fiber: 7 g
- Sugars: 24 g
- Fat: 3 g
- Saturated Fat: 0.5 g

- Cholesterol: 0 mg
- Sodium: 60 mg
- Potassium: 700 mg
- Vitamin A: 6700 IU
- Vitamin C: 80 mg
- Calcium: 100 mg
- Iron: 1.5 mg

Directions

- Soak the Chia Seeds: In a small bowl, soak the chia seeds in a quarter cup of water for about 5-10 minutes, until they expand and form a gel-like consistency.
- Prepare the Ingredients: Peel and cube the mango. Wash and chop the kale leaves, removing the tough stems.
- Blending: In a blender, combine the soaked chia seeds, mango cubes, chopped kale, and coconut water. Add ice cubes for a colder smoothie.
- Blending Speed and Time: Blend on high speed for about 60-90 seconds, until the smoothie is smooth and the kale is thoroughly blended.
- Taste and Adjust: If the smoothie is too thick, add more coconut water. If you prefer it sweeter, add a small amount of agave syrup or maple syrup.
- Serve Immediately: Pour into glasses and enjoy your nourishing "Chia Fresh Kick" smoothie!

Tips and Techniques

- Ingredient Alternatives: If mango is not available, you can use pineapple or papaya for a similar tropical flavor. Spinach can be used in place of kale for a milder taste.
- Nutrition Boost: Add a scoop of your favorite plant-based protein powder for an extra protein kick.
- Storage: This smoothie is best enjoyed fresh, but it can be stored in the refrigerator for up to 24 hours. Stir well before drinking.
- The "Chia Fresh Kick" smoothie is a wonderful way to enjoy a blend of superfoods, offering a perfect mix of taste and nutrition!

Cocoa Avocado Bliss Vegan Smoothie

Ingredients

- Avocado: 1/2 medium, pitted and scooped
- Banana: 1 medium, ripe
- Raw cocoa powder: 2 tablespoons
- Oat milk: 1 cup (unsweetened, to keep it vegan-friendly)
- Ice cubes: a handful (optional)

Nutritional Info

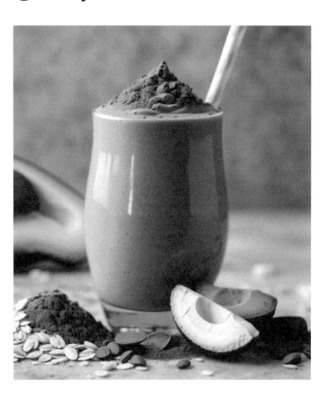

- Calories: 280 kcal
- Protein: 5 g
- Carbohydrates: 37 g
- Dietary Fiber: 9 g
- Sugars: 15 g
- Fat: 15 g
- Saturated Fat: 2.5 g
- Cholesterol: 0 mg
- Sodium: 60 mg
- Potassium: 850 mg
- Vitamin C: 15 mg
- Calcium: 200 mg
- Iron: 2 mg

Directions

- Prepare the Ingredients: Halve the avocado, remove the pit, and scoop out the flesh. Peel the banana.
- Blending: In a blender, add the avocado, banana, raw cocoa powder, and oat milk. Include ice cubes if you want a colder smoothie.
- Blending Speed and Time: Blend on high speed for about 60 seconds, or until the mixture is smooth and creamy.
- Taste and Adjust: If the smoothie is too thick, add more oat milk. For added sweetness, you can add a teaspoon of agave syrup or maple syrup.
- Serve Immediately: Pour into glasses and enjoy your luxurious "Cocoa Avocado Bliss" smoothie!

Tips and Techniques

- Ingredient Alternatives: If oat milk is not available, you can use any other plant-based milk, such as almond or soy milk. For an extra protein boost, consider adding a scoop of your favorite plant-based protein powder.
- Nutrition Boost: To enhance the nutritional value, you can add a tablespoon of chia seeds or hemp seeds.
- Storage: This smoothie is best enjoyed fresh, but it can be stored in the refrigerator for up to 24 hours. Give it a good stir or shake before consuming.
- The "Cocoa Avocado Bliss" smoothie is a fantastic choice for anyone seeking a delicious, heart-healthy, and indulgent vegan beverage!

Sunset Beet Mix Vegan Smoothie

Ingredients

- Beetroot: 1 small, cooked and peeled (about 100g)
- Orange: 1 medium, peeled and segmented
- Carrot: 1 medium, peeled and chopped
- Lemon juice: from 1/2 medium lemon
- Water or coconut water: 1 cup (240ml)
- Ice cubes: a handful (optional)

Nutritional Info

- Calories: 150 kcal
- Protein: 3 g
- Carbohydrates: 35 g
- Dietary Fiber: 8 g
- Sugars: 25 g
- Fat: 0.5 g
- Saturated Fat: 0 g

- Cholesterol: 0 mg
- Sodium: 120 mg
- Potassium: 700 mg
- Vitamin A: 11000 IU
- Vitamin C: 70 mg
- Calcium: 60 mg
- Iron: 1.5 mg

⏱ Preparation Time: 10m

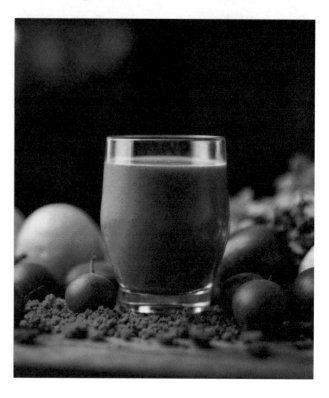

Directions

- Prepare the Ingredients: If using a fresh beetroot, cook it until tender, then peel and chop. Peel and segment the orange. Peel and chop the carrot. Squeeze the lemon for juice.
- Blending: In a blender, combine the cooked beetroot, orange segments, chopped carrot, lemon juice, and water or coconut water. Add ice cubes for a chilled smoothie.
- Blending Speed and Time: Blend on high speed for about 60-90 seconds, until the smoothie is smooth and all ingredients are fully blended.
- Taste and Adjust: If the smoothie is too thick, add more water or coconut water. Adjust the sweetness or tartness as needed, potentially adding a small amount of agave syrup or more lemon juice.
- Serve Immediately: Pour into glasses and enjoy your vibrant and nutritious "Sunset Beet Mix" smoothie!

Tips and Techniques

- Ingredient Alternatives: If fresh beetroot is not available, you can use pre-cooked packaged beets. If you prefer a sweeter smoothie, consider adding an apple or a banana.
- Nutrition Boost: Add a tablespoon of ground flaxseed or chia seeds for extra fiber and omega-3 fatty acids.
- Storage: Best consumed fresh. However, if needed, it can be stored in the refrigerator for up to 24 hours. Stir well before drinking.
- The "Sunset Beet Mix" smoothie is a fantastic way to enjoy the natural flavors of vegetables and fruits in a delicious, healthy drink!

Cucumber Melon Cooler Vegan Smoothie

Ingredients

- Cucumber: 1 medium, peeled and chopped (about 150g)
- Honeydew melon: 1 cup, cubed (about 170g)
- Fresh mint leaves: 1/4 cup (about 15g)
- Almond milk: 1 cup (unsweetened)
- Ice cubes: a handful (optional)

🕐 Preparation Time: 10m

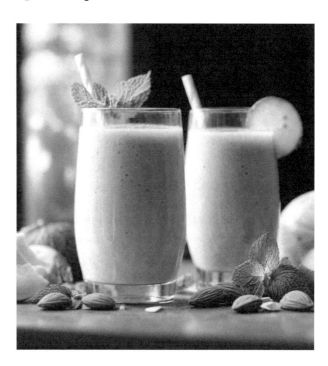

Nutritional Info

- Calories: 100 kcal
- Protein: 2 g
- Carbohydrates: 20 g
- Dietary Fiber: 2 g
- Sugars: 15 g
- Fat: 2.5 g
- Saturated Fat: 0 g

- Cholesterol: 0 mg
- Sodium: 180 mg
- Potassium: 400 mg
- Vitamin C: 20 mg
- Calcium: 300 mg
- Iron: 0.5 mg

Directions

- Prepare the Ingredients: Peel and chop the cucumber. Cube the honeydew melon. Rinse the mint leaves.
- Blending: In a blender, combine the cucumber, honeydew melon, mint leaves, and almond milk. Add ice cubes if you want a cooler smoothie.
- Blending Speed and Time: Blend on high speed for about 60 seconds, or until the mixture is smooth.
- Taste and Adjust: If the smoothie is too thick, add more almond milk. If you prefer it sweeter, consider adding a teaspoon of agave syrup.
- Serve Immediately: Pour into glasses and enjoy your refreshing "Cucumber Melon Cooler" smoothie!

Tips and Techniques

- Ingredient Alternatives: If honeydew melon is not available, you can use cantaloupe or watermelon for a similar refreshing taste. If almond milk is not available, any other plant-based milk like soy or oat milk can be used.
- Nutrition Boost: For added nutrients, consider including a tablespoon of chia seeds or a handful of spinach.
- Storage: This smoothie is best enjoyed fresh. However, if needed, it can be stored in the refrigerator for a few hours.
- The "Cucumber Melon Cooler" is a perfect choice for anyone looking for a hydrating, nutritious, and delicious vegan smoothie!

Golden Flax Elixir Vegan Smoothie

Ingredients

- Ground flaxseeds: 2 tablespoons
- Banana: 1 medium, ripe
- Peach slices: 1 cup (fresh or frozen)
- Soy milk: 1 cup (unsweetened, to keep it vegan-friendly)
- Ice cubes: a handful (optional, especially if using frozen peach slices)

Nutritional Info

- Calories: 250 kcal
- Protein: 8 g
- Carbohydrates: 38 g
- Dietary Fiber: 7 g
- Sugars: 20 g
- Fat: 8 g
- Saturated Fat: 1 g
- Cholesterol: 0 mg
- Sodium: 90 mg
- Potassium: 600 mg
- Vitamin C: 10 mg
- Calcium: 300 mg
- Iron: 2 mg

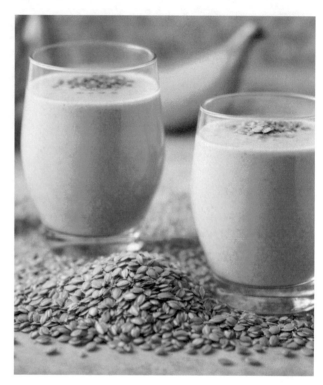

⏱ Preparation Time: 10m

Directions

- Prepare the Ingredients: Peel the banana. If using fresh peaches, wash, pit, and slice them.
- Blending: In a blender, add the ground flaxseeds, banana, peach slices, and soy milk. Include ice cubes if you prefer a colder smoothie.
- Blending Speed and Time: Blend on high speed for about 60 seconds, or until the mixture is smooth and creamy.
- Taste and Adjust: If the smoothie is too thick, add more soy milk. If you prefer additional sweetness, add a teaspoon of agave syrup or maple syrup.
- Serve Immediately: Pour into glasses and enjoy your "Golden Flax Elixir" smoothie!

Tips and Techniques

- Ingredient Alternatives: If soy milk is not available, you can use any other plant-based milk, such as almond or oat milk. If peaches are not in season, you can substitute them with nectarines or mangoes for a similar flavor profile.
- Nutrition Boost: For an extra protein kick, add a scoop of your favorite plant-based protein powder.
- Storage: This smoothie is best enjoyed fresh, but it can be stored in the refrigerator for up to 24 hours. Stir well before drinking.
- The "Golden Flax Elixir" smoothie is a great way to enjoy a delicious, healthy blend of fruits and flaxseeds, perfect for a vegan diet!

Pumpkin Spice Medley Vegan

Ingredients

- Pumpkin puree: 1/2 cup (canned or homemade, ensure it's pure pumpkin without additives)
- Cinnamon: 1/2 teaspoon
- Nutmeg: 1/4 teaspoon
- Vanilla almond milk: 1 cup (unsweetened)
- Ice cubes: a handful (optional)
- Optional sweetener: Maple syrup or agave syrup, to taste (optional)

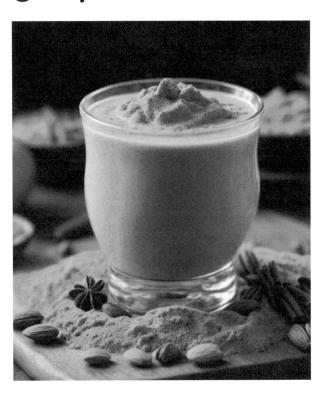

Nutritional Info

- Calories: 120 kcal
- Protein: 2 g
- Carbohydrates: 24 g
- Dietary Fiber: 5 g
- Sugars: 12 g
- Fat: 2.5 g
- Saturated Fat: 0 g
- Cholesterol: 0 mg
- Sodium: 180 mg
- Potassium: 250 mg
- Vitamin A: 15000 IU
- Vitamin C: 4 mg
- Calcium: 300 mg
- Iron: 1.5 mg

Directions

- Prepare the Ingredients: If using homemade pumpkin puree, prepare it in advance.
- Blending: In a blender, combine the pumpkin puree, cinnamon, nutmeg, and vanilla almond milk. Add ice cubes for a chilled smoothie.
- Blending Speed and Time: Blend on high speed for about 60 seconds, or until the mixture is smooth and creamy.
- Taste and Adjust: If the smoothie is too thick, add more almond milk. Adjust sweetness with maple syrup or agave syrup, if desired.
- Serve Immediately: Pour into glasses and enjoy your delicious "Pumpkin Spice Medley" smoothie!

Tips and Techniques

- Ingredient Alternatives: If vanilla almond milk is not available, you can use plain almond milk with a splash of vanilla extract. For a richer smoothie, add a banana.
- Nutrition Boost: To add protein, include a scoop of your favorite plant-based protein powder.
- Storage: This smoothie is best enjoyed fresh, but it can be refrigerated for up to 24 hours. Stir well before drinking.
- The "Pumpkin Spice Medley" smoothie is a wonderful way to enjoy the flavors of the season in a healthy, vegan-friendly drink!

Pear Ginger Harmony Vegan Smoothie

Ingredients

- Pear: 1 large, ripe, cored and chopped
- Fresh ginger: 1-inch piece, peeled and grated
- Spinach: 1 cup, fresh
- Flaxseed milk: 1 cup (unsweetened, to keep it vegan-friendly)
- Ice cubes: a handful (optional)

🕐 Preparation Time: 10m

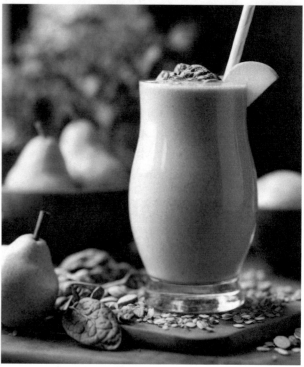

Nutritional Info

- Calories: 150 kcal
- Protein: 3 g
- Carbohydrates: 30 g
- Dietary Fiber: 6 g
- Sugars: 20 g
- Fat: 3 g
- Saturated Fat: 0 g
- Cholesterol: 0 mg
- Sodium: 80 mg
- Potassium: 400 mg
- Vitamin A: 2900 IU
- Vitamin C: 20 mg
- Calcium: 300 mg
- Iron: 1.5 mg

Directions

- Prepare the Ingredients: Wash and chop the pear. Peel and grate the ginger. Rinse the spinach leaves.
- Blending: In a blender, combine the chopped pear, grated ginger, spinach, and flaxseed milk. Add ice cubes if you prefer a colder smoothie.
- Blending Speed and Time: Blend on high speed for about 60 seconds, or until the mixture is smooth and creamy.
- Taste and Adjust: If the smoothie is too thick, add more flaxseed milk. If you prefer it sweeter, consider adding a teaspoon of agave syrup or maple syrup.
- Serve Immediately: Pour into glasses and enjoy your refreshing "Pear Ginger Harmony" smoothie!

Tips and Techniques

- Ingredient Alternatives: If flaxseed milk is not available, you can use any other plant-based milk, such as almond or soy milk. For added sweetness, you can include a banana.
- Nutrition Boost: To enhance the nutritional value, you can add a tablespoon of chia seeds or a scoop of your favorite plant-based protein powder.
- Storage: This smoothie is best enjoyed fresh, but it can be refrigerated for up to 24 hours. Stir well before drinking.

Matcha Green Tea Vegan Smoothie

Ingredients

- Matcha green tea powder: 1 teaspoon
- Banana: 1 medium, ripe
- Spinach: 1 cup, fresh
- Coconut water: 1 cup (ensure it's pure and without added sugars for a vegan option)
- Ice cubes: a handful (optional)

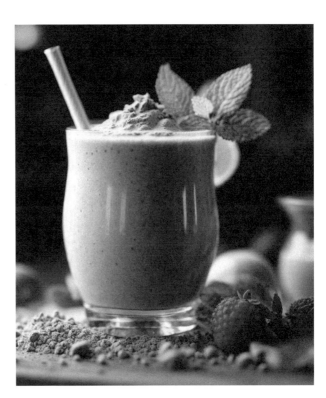

Nutritional Info

- Calories: 150 kcal
- Protein: 3 g
- Carbohydrates: 35 g
- Dietary Fiber: 5 g
- Sugars: 20 g
- Fat: 0.5 g
- Saturated Fat: 0 g

- Cholesterol: 0 mg
- Sodium: 250 mg
- Potassium: 850 mg
- Vitamin A: 2900 IU
- Vitamin C: 30 mg
- Calcium: 60 mg
- Iron: 2 mg

Directions

- Prepare the Ingredients: Peel the banana. Rinse the spinach leaves.
- Blending: In a blender, combine the matcha green tea powder, banana, spinach, and coconut water. Add ice cubes if you prefer a chilled smoothie.
- Blending Speed and Time: Blend on high speed for about 60 seconds, or until the mixture is smooth and the spinach is fully blended.
- Taste and Adjust: If the smoothie is too thick, add more coconut water. If you prefer it sweeter, you can add a teaspoon of agave syrup or maple syrup.
- Serve Immediately: Pour into glasses and enjoy your vibrant and healthy "Matcha Green Tea Magic" smoothie!

Tips and Techniques

- Ingredient Alternatives: If coconut water is not available, you can use almond milk or another plant-based milk. Adding a pear or an apple can enhance the sweetness and texture.
- Nutrition Boost: For extra protein and healthy fats, include a tablespoon of chia seeds or a scoop of your favorite plant-based protein powder.
- Storage: This smoothie is best enjoyed fresh. However, it can be stored in the refrigerator for up to 24 hours. Stir well before drinking.
- The "Matcha Green Tea Magic" smoothie is a delightful way to enjoy the benefits of matcha in a delicious, vegan-friendly drink!

CHAPTER 5

Post-Workout Power Blends

Post-Workout Citrus Hydrator Smoothie

Ingredients

- Oranges: 2 medium, peeled and segmented
- Carrot: 1 large, peeled and chopped
- Fresh ginger: 1-inch piece, peeled and grated
- Unflavored protein powder: 1 scoop
- Water or coconut water: 1 cup
- Ice cubes: a handful (optional)

Nutritional Info

- Calories: 200-250 kcal
- Protein: 15-20 g
- Carbohydrates: 30-35 g
- Dietary Fiber: 5-6 g
- Sugars: 20-25 g
- Fat: 1-2 g
- Saturated Fat: 0 g
- Cholesterol: 0-10 mg
- Sodium: 100-150 mg
- Potassium: 600-700 mg
- Vitamin C: 100 mg
- Calcium: 100-150 mg
- Iron: 1 mg

Directions

- Prepare the Ingredients: Peel and segment the oranges, ensuring to remove any seeds and pith. Peel and chop the carrot. Peel and grate the ginger.
- Blending: In a blender, combine the orange segments, chopped carrot, grated ginger, unflavored protein powder, and water or coconut water. Add ice cubes for a cooler smoothie.
- Blending Speed and Time: Blend on high speed for about 60 seconds, or until the smoothie is smooth and creamy.
- Taste and Adjust: If the smoothie is too thick, add more water or coconut water. If you prefer it sweeter, you can add a small amount of honey or agave syrup.
- Serve Immediately: Pour into glasses and enjoy your refreshing Post-Workout Citrus Hydrator smoothie!

Tips and Techniques

- Ingredient Alternatives: If you prefer a sweeter taste, you can add an apple or a pear. If unflavored protein powder isn't available, vanilla protein powder can be used as an alternative.
- Nutrition Boost: Add a handful of spinach or kale for added vitamins and minerals without significantly altering the taste.
- Storage: Best consumed immediately. However, if necessary, it can be stored in the refrigerator for up to 24 hours. Stir well before drinking.
- The Post-Workout Citrus Hydrator smoothie is a perfect choice for a delicious, nutrient-rich drink that helps in rehydration and muscle recovery after a workout!

Muscle Recovery Mango Smoothie

Ingredients

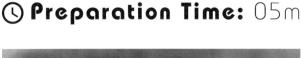
- Mango: 1 cup, cubed (fresh or frozen)
- Greek yogurt: 1/2 cup (plain, non-fat)
- Whey protein powder: 1 scoop (flavor of choice)
- Turmeric: 1/4 teaspoon
- Water or almond milk: 1/2 cup
- Ice cubes: a handful (optional, if using fresh mango)

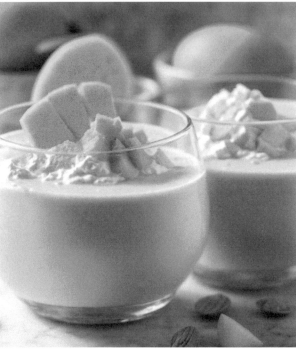

Nutritional Info

- Calories: 250-300 kcal
- Protein: 20-25 g
- Carbohydrates: 35-40 g
- Dietary Fiber: 3 g
- Sugars: 28 g
- Fat: 1 g
- Saturated Fat: 0 g
- Cholesterol: 10 mg
- Sodium: 100 mg
- Potassium: 500 mg
- Vitamin A: 1000 IU
- Vitamin C: 60 mg
- Calcium: 200 mg
- Iron: 1 mg

Directions

- Prepare the Ingredients: If using fresh mango, peel and cube it. Measure the Greek yogurt, whey protein powder, and turmeric.
- Blending: In a blender, combine the mango, Greek yogurt, whey protein powder, turmeric, and water or almond milk. Add ice cubes if using fresh mango.
- Blending Speed and Time: Blend on high speed for about 60 seconds, or until the mixture is smooth and creamy.
- Taste and Adjust: If the smoothie is too thick, add more liquid. If you prefer more sweetness, you can add a teaspoon of honey or agave syrup.
- Serve Immediately: Pour into a glass and enjoy your refreshing and rejuvenating Muscle Recovery Mango Tango smoothie!

Tips and Techniques

- Ingredient Alternatives: If you're lactose intolerant or prefer a plant-based option, you can substitute Greek yogurt with a dairy-free yogurt and whey protein with a plant-based protein powder.
- Nutrition Boost: For added fiber and omega-3 fatty acids, include a tablespoon of chia seeds or flaxseeds.
- Storage: This smoothie is best enjoyed fresh to maximize the benefits of the ingredients, particularly the whey protein and turmeric.
- The Muscle Recovery Mango Tango is an excellent choice for a post-workout drink, providing the necessary nutrients to aid in muscle recovery and reduce inflammation.

Berry Protein Powerhouse Smoothie

Ingredients

🕐 **Preparation Time:** 05m

- Mixed berries (strawberries, blueberries, raspberries, blackberries): 1 cup, fresh or frozen
- Spinach: 1 cup, fresh
- Plant-based protein powder: 1 scoop (flavor of your choice, although vanilla or unflavored works well)
- Almond milk: 1 cup (unsweetened)

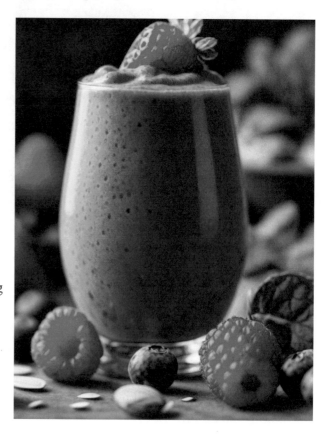

Nutritional Info

- Calories: 200-250 kcal
- Protein: 15-20 g
- Carbohydrates: 25-30 g
- Dietary Fiber: 5 g
- Sugars: 10-15 g
- Fat: 3-5 g
- Saturated Fat: 0 g
- Cholesterol: 0 mg
- Sodium: 150-200 mg
- Potassium: 400-500 mg
- Vitamin A: 2900 IU
- Vitamin C: 60 mg
- Calcium: 300-400 mg
- Iron: 2-3 mg

Directions

- Prepare the Ingredients: If using fresh berries, wash them thoroughly. Rinse the spinach leaves.
- Blending: In a blender, combine the mixed berries, spinach, plant-based protein powder, and almond milk.
- Blending Speed and Time: Blend on high speed for about 60 seconds, or until the smoothie is smooth and creamy.
- Taste and Adjust: If the smoothie is too thick, add a bit more almond milk. Adjust the sweetness to your preference, if necessary, with a natural sweetener like stevia or agave syrup.
- Serve Immediately: Pour into a glass and enjoy your delicious Berry Protein Powerhouse smoothie!

Tips and Techniques

- Ingredient Alternatives: If you don't have almond milk, any other plant-based milk like soy or oat milk can be used. For added nutrition, consider including a tablespoon of chia seeds or flaxseeds.
- Nutrition Boost: Add a handful of kale or a tablespoon of nut butter for extra nutrients and healthy fats.
- Storage: Best consumed immediately. However, if needed, it can be stored in the refrigerator for up to 24 hours. Stir well before drinking.
- The Berry Protein Powerhouse smoothie is a fantastic way to get a delicious, protein-packed, and healthy vegan drink!

Peanut Butter Power Play Smoothie

Ingredients

- Creamy peanut butter: 2 tablespoons
- Banana: 1 medium, ripe
- Oat milk: 1 cup (unsweetened)
- Chocolate protein powder: 1 scoop
- Ice cubes: a handful (optional, especially if using a frozen banana)

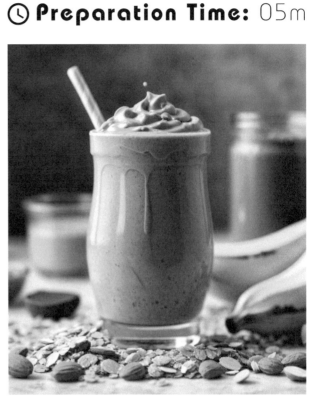

Nutritional Info

- Calories: 350-400 kcal
- Protein: 20-25 g
- Carbohydrates: 40-45 g
- Dietary Fiber: 5 g
- Sugars: 20 g
- Fat: 15-18 g
- Saturated Fat: 3-4 g
- Cholesterol: 0-10 mg
- Sodium: 200-250 mg
- Potassium: 600-700 mg
- Vitamin C: 10 mg
- Calcium: 300-350 mg
- Iron: 2 mg

Directions

- Prepare the Ingredients: Peel the banana. Measure the peanut butter, oat milk, and chocolate protein powder.
- Blending: In a blender, combine the peanut butter, banana, oat milk, and chocolate protein powder. Add ice cubes if you prefer a colder smoothie.
- Blending Speed and Time: Blend on high speed for about 60 seconds, or until the smoothie is smooth and creamy.
- Taste and Adjust: If the smoothie is too thick, add more oat milk. If you prefer more sweetness, consider adding a teaspoon of honey or maple syrup.
- Serve Immediately: Pour into a glass and enjoy your rich and energizing Peanut Butter Power Play smoothie!

Tips and Techniques

- Ingredient Alternatives: If you're allergic to peanuts, you can use almond butter or sunflower seed butter as an alternative. If oat milk is not available, any other plant-based milk like soy or almond milk can be used.
- Nutrition Boost: For added fiber and omega-3 fatty acids, include a tablespoon of ground flaxseeds or chia seeds.
- Storage: This smoothie is best enjoyed fresh, but it can be refrigerated for up to 24 hours. Stir well before drinking.
- This smoothie is a perfect combination of delicious flavors, making it an excellent choice!

Cherry Almond Recharge Smoothie

Ingredients

- Tart cherries: 1 cup, fresh or frozen
- Almond butter: 2 tablespoons
- Vanilla protein powder: 1 scoop
- Coconut water: 1 cup (without added sugars)
- Ice cubes: a handful (optional, but recommended if using fresh cherries)

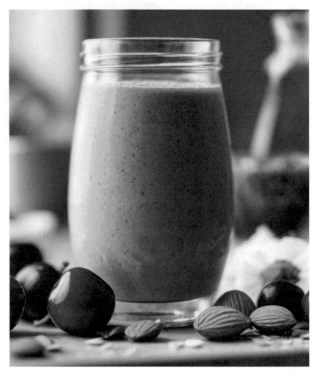

Nutritional Info

- Calories: 350-400 kcal
- Protein: 15-20 g
- Carbohydrates: 35-40 g
- Dietary Fiber: 4 g
- Sugars: 20-25 g
- Fat: 15-18 g
- Saturated Fat: 2-3 g
- Cholesterol: 0-10 mg
- Sodium: 150-200 mg
- Potassium: 600-700 mg
- Vitamin C: 15 mg
- Calcium: 200-250 mg
- Iron: 2 mg

Directions

- Prepare the Ingredients: If using frozen cherries, measure out one cup. Measure the almond butter and vanilla protein powder. Ensure the coconut water is ready to use.
- Blending: In a blender, combine the tart cherries, almond butter, vanilla protein powder, and coconut water. Add ice cubes if using fresh cherries.
- Blending Speed and Time: Blend on high speed for about 60 seconds, or until the smoothie is smooth and creamy.
- Taste and Adjust: If the smoothie is too thick, add more coconut water. Adjust the sweetness if necessary, perhaps with a bit of honey or agave syrup.
- Serve Immediately: Pour into glasses and enjoy your refreshing Cherry Almond Recharge smoothie!

Tips and Techniques

- Ingredient Alternatives: If almond butter is not available, you can use peanut butter or cashew butter. If coconut water is not to your liking, almond milk can be a suitable substitute.
- Nutrition Boost: For added antioxidants and fiber, include a tablespoon of ground flaxseeds or chia seeds.
- Storage: This smoothie is best enjoyed fresh, but it can be stored in the refrigerator for up to 24 hours. Give it a good shake before drinking.
- The Cherry Almond Recharge smoothie is a fantastic way to enjoy a delicious, nutrient-rich drink that's perfect for recharging your energy!

Green Muscle Machine Smoothie

Ingredients

- Kale: 1 cup, stems removed and chopped
- Banana: 1 medium, ripe
- Hemp seeds: 2 tablespoons
- Almond milk: 1 cup (unsweetened)
- Vanilla protein powder: 1 scoop
- Ice cubes: a handful (optional, recommended if the banana isn't frozen)

Nutritional Info

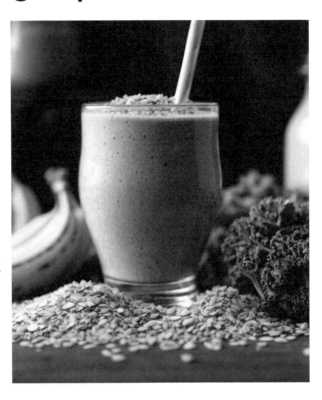

- Calories: 300-350 kcal
- Protein: 20-25 g
- Carbohydrates: 35-40 g
- Dietary Fiber: 5-6 g
- Sugars: 15-20 g
- Fat: 9-11 g
- Saturated Fat: 1-2 g

- Cholesterol: 0-10 mg
- Sodium: 150-200 mg
- Potassium: 600-700 mg
- Vitamin A: 6700 IU
- Vitamin C: 80 mg
- Calcium: 300-350 mg
- Iron: 3-4 mg

Directions

- Prepare the Ingredients: Wash and chop the kale leaves, removing the stems. Peel the banana. Measure the hemp seeds, almond milk, and vanilla protein powder.
- Blending: In a blender, combine the kale, banana, hemp seeds, almond milk, and vanilla protein powder. Add ice cubes if the banana isn't frozen.
- Blending Speed and Time: Blend on high speed for about 60 seconds, or until the smoothie is smooth and creamy.
- Taste and Adjust: If the smoothie is too thick, add more almond milk. Adjust sweetness if necessary, perhaps with a bit of honey or agave syrup (if not using a sweetened protein powder).
- Serve Immediately: Pour into a glass and enjoy your nutrient-packed Green Muscle Machine smoothie!

Tips and Techniques

- Ingredient Alternatives: If almond milk is not available, any plant-based milk like soy or oat milk can be used. If kale is not to your liking, spinach is a great alternative.
- Nutrition Boost: For added omega-3 fatty acids, you can include a tablespoon of ground flaxseeds or chia seeds.
- Storage: Best consumed immediately for maximum freshness and nutrient retention. However, if needed, it can be stored in the refrigerator for up to 24 hours. Stir well before drinking.
- The Green Muscle Machine smoothie is a fantastic choice for anyone looking for a delicious, nourishing post-workout drink that supports muscle recovery and overall health!

Blueberry Quinoa Boost Smoothie

Ingredients

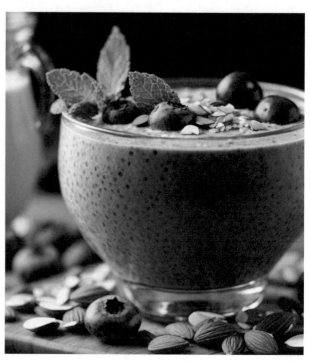

- Blueberries: 1 cup, fresh or frozen
- Cooked quinoa: 1/2 cup (cooled)
- Greek yogurt: 1/2 cup (plain, non-fat)
- Almond milk: 1/2 cup (unsweetened)
- Ice cubes: a handful (optional, recommended if using fresh blueberries)

🕐 Preparation Time: 10m

Nutritional Info

- Calories: 250-300 kcal
- Protein: 10-15 g
- Carbohydrates: 40-45 g
- Dietary Fiber: 5-6 g
- Sugars: 15-20 g
- Fat: 3-5 g
- Saturated Fat: 0.5 g
- Cholesterol: 5 mg
- Sodium: 100-150 mg
- Potassium: 400-500 mg
- Vitamin C: 15 mg
- Calcium: 200-250 mg
- Iron: 1.5 mg

Directions

- Prepare the Ingredients: If using fresh blueberries, wash them thoroughly. Ensure the quinoa is cooked, cooled, and ready to use. Measure the Greek yogurt and almond milk.
- Blending: In a blender, combine the blueberries, cooked quinoa, Greek yogurt, and almond milk. Add ice cubes if using fresh blueberries.
- Blending Speed and Time: Blend on high speed for about 60 seconds, or until the smoothie is smooth and creamy.
- Taste and Adjust: If the smoothie is too thick, add more almond milk. If you prefer additional sweetness, consider adding a teaspoon of honey or agave syrup.
- Serve Immediately: Pour into a glass and enjoy your nutritious Blueberry Quinoa Boost smoothie!

Tips and Techniques

- Ingredient Alternatives: If Greek yogurt is not available, you can use any plain yogurt or a plant-based yogurt alternative. If almond milk is not to your liking, you can use any other plant-based milk like soy or oat milk.
- Nutrition Boost: For added antioxidants and omega-3 fatty acids, include a tablespoon of ground flaxseeds or chia seeds.
- Storage: Best consumed immediately. However, if necessary, it can be stored in the refrigerator for up to 24 hours. Stir well before drinking.
- The Blueberry Quinoa Boost smoothie is a perfect combination of taste and nutrition, making it an excellent choice for post-workout recovery and overall health!

Fig and Date Recovery Smoothie

Ingredients

- Dried figs: 3-4, stems removed
- Dates: 3-4, pitted
- Almond milk: 1 cup (unsweetened)
- Cinnamon: 1/2 teaspoon
- Protein powder: 1 scoop

Nutritional Info

- Calories: 300-350 kcal
- Protein: 15-20 g
- Carbohydrates: 50-55 g
- Dietary Fiber: 6-7 g
- Sugars: 40-45 g
- Fat: 3-5 g
- Saturated Fat: 0 g
- Cholesterol: 0-10 mg
- Sodium: 100-150 mg
- Potassium: 600-700 mg
- Vitamin A: 100 IU
- Vitamin C: 1 mg
- Calcium: 300-350 mg
- Iron: 2 mg

⏱ Preparation Time: 10m

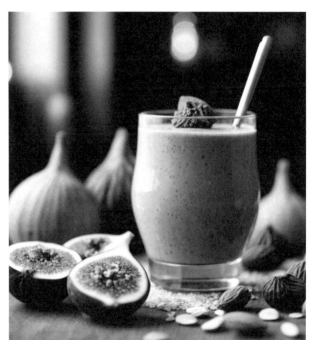

Directions

- Prepare the Ingredients: Remove the stems from the dried figs and pits from the dates. If the dried figs and dates are very hard, you can soak them in warm water for about 10 minutes to soften.
- Blending: In a blender, combine the softened figs, dates, almond milk, cinnamon, and protein powder.
- Blending Speed and Time: Blend on high speed for about 60 seconds, or until the smoothie is smooth and creamy.
- Taste and Adjust: If the smoothie is too thick, add more almond milk. If you prefer it sweeter, the natural sweetness from the figs and dates should be sufficient, but you can add a bit of honey or maple syrup if needed.
- Serve Immediately: Pour into glasses and enjoy your Fig and Date Recovery Blend smoothie!

Tips and Techniques

- Ingredient Alternatives: If almond milk is not available, you can use any other plant-based milk like soy or oat milk. If you're not a fan of cinnamon, you can omit it or replace it with vanilla extract.
- Nutrition Boost: Add a tablespoon of chia seeds or flaxseeds for added omega-3 fatty acids and fiber.
- Storage: Best consumed immediately. However, if necessary, it can be stored in the refrigerator for up to 24 hours. Stir well before drinking.
- The Fig and Date Recovery Blend smoothie is a superb choice for a post-workout drink, offering a delicious way to replenish energy and aid in muscle recovery!

CHAPTER 6
Energizing Smoothie For a Morning Boost

🕐 **Preparation Time:** 05m

Cacao Power Smoothie

Ingredients

- Raw cacao powder: 2 tablespoons
- Banana: 1 medium, ripe
- Peanut butter: 2 tablespoons
- Soy milk: 1 cup (unsweetened)

Nutritional Info

- Calories: 350-400 kcal
- Protein: 15-20 g
- Carbohydrates: 40-45 g
- Dietary Fiber: 5-6 g
- Sugars: 20-25 g
- Fat: 18-20 g
- Saturated Fat: 4-5 g
- Cholesterol: 0 mg
- Sodium: 200-250 mg
- Potassium: 700-800 mg
- Vitamin C: 10 mg
- Calcium: 300-350 mg
- Iron: 3-4 mg

Directions

- Prepare the Ingredients: Peel the banana.
- Blending: In a blender, combine the raw cacao powder, banana, peanut butter, and soy milk.
- Blending Speed and Time: Blend on high speed for about 60 seconds, or until the smoothie is smooth and creamy.
- Taste and Adjust: If the smoothie is too thick, add more soy milk. If you prefer it sweeter, consider adding a teaspoon of honey or agave syrup.
- Serve Immediately: Pour into glasses and enjoy your rich and energizing Cacao Power Smoothie!

Tips and Techniques

- Ingredient Alternatives: If you're allergic to peanuts, almond butter or sunflower seed butter can be used as an alternative. If soy milk is not to your liking, any other plant-based milk like almond or oat milk can be used.
- Nutrition Boost: For added protein, include a scoop of your favorite protein powder. You can also add a tablespoon of chia seeds or flaxseeds for extra fiber and omega-3 fatty acids.
- Storage: Best consumed immediately. However, if necessary, it can be stored in the refrigerator for up to 24 hours. Stir well before drinking.
- The Cacao Power Smoothie is a delightful and nutritious way to start your day, offering a delicious blend of flavors and a boost of energy!

Berry Awake Smoothie

Ingredients

- Mixed berries (such as strawberries, blueberries, raspberries): 1 cup, fresh or frozen
- Banana: 1 medium, ripe
- Greek yogurt: 1/2 cup (plain, non-fat or low-fat)
- Orange juice: 1/4 cup (freshly squeezed for the best flavor)

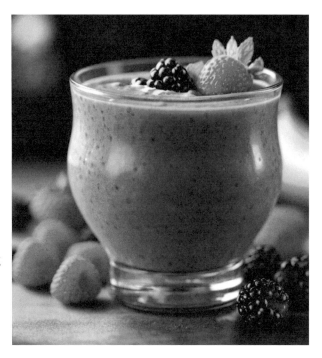

Nutritional Info

- Calories: 200-250 kcal
- Protein: 10-15 g
- Carbohydrates: 40-45 g
- Dietary Fiber: 5-6 g
- Sugars: 25-30 g
- Fat: 0.5-1 g
- Saturated Fat: 0 g
- Cholesterol: 5 mg
- Sodium: 50-70 mg
- Potassium: 500-600 mg
- Vitamin C: 60-70 mg
- Calcium: 150-200 mg
- Iron: 1 mg

Directions

- Prepare the Ingredients: If using fresh berries, wash them thoroughly. Peel the banana.
- Blending: In a blender, combine the mixed berries, banana, Greek yogurt, and orange juice.
- Blending Speed and Time: Blend on high speed for about 60 seconds, or until the smoothie is smooth and creamy.
- Taste and Adjust: If the smoothie is too thick, add a bit more orange juice or water. If you prefer it sweeter, consider adding a teaspoon of honey or agave syrup.
- Serve Immediately: Pour into glasses and enjoy your refreshing Berry Awake Smoothie!

Tips and Techniques

- Ingredient Alternatives: If Greek yogurt is not available, any plain yogurt will work. For a vegan option, use a plant-based yogurt and substitute orange juice with plant-based milk if preferred.
- Nutrition Boost: Add a tablespoon of chia seeds or ground flaxseeds for extra fiber and omega-3 fatty acids.
- Storage: This smoothie is best enjoyed fresh. However, if necessary, it can be stored in the refrigerator for up to 24 hours. Stir well before drinking.
- The Berry Awake Smoothie is a perfect choice for an energizing and nutritious start to your day!

Red Berry Refresher Smoothie

Ingredients

⏱ Preparation Time: 10m

- Strawberries: 1 cup, fresh or frozen
- Raspberries: 1/2 cup, fresh or frozen
- Beetroot: 1 small, cooked and peeled (or raw if you have a powerful blender)
- Orange juice: 1 cup (freshly squeezed for the best flavor)

Nutritional Info

- Calories: 150-200 kcal
- Protein: 2-3 g
- Carbohydrates: 35-40 g
- Dietary Fiber: 6-7 g
- Sugars: 25-30 g
- Fat: 0.5 g
- Saturated Fat: 0 g
- Cholesterol: 0 mg
- Sodium: 50-70 mg
- Potassium: 500-600 mg
- Vitamin C: 90-100 mg
- Calcium: 40-50 mg
- Iron: 1-1.5 mg

Directions

- Prepare the Ingredients: If using fresh berries, wash them thoroughly. If you're using cooked beetroot, make sure it's cooled and peeled. If using raw beetroot, peel and chop it.
- Blending: In a blender, combine the strawberries, raspberries, beetroot, and orange juice.
- Blending Speed and Time: Blend on high speed for about 60 seconds, or until the smoothie is smooth and creamy.
- Taste and Adjust: If the smoothie is too thick, add more orange juice. If you prefer it sweeter, consider adding a bit of honey or agave syrup.
- Serve Immediately: Pour into glasses and enjoy your vibrant and energizing Red Berry Refresher smoothie!

Tips and Techniques

- Ingredient Alternatives: If you don't have raspberries, you can use more strawberries or even blueberries. If fresh orange juice is not available, you can use store-bought, but check for added sugars.
- Nutrition Boost: Add a tablespoon of chia seeds or ground flaxseed for added fiber and omega-3 fatty acids.
- Storage: Best consumed immediately. However, if necessary, it can be stored in the refrigerator for up to 24 hours. Stir well before drinking.
- The Red Berry Refresher smoothie is a perfect way to start your day with a burst of freshness and a boost of energy!

Espresso Energy Booster Smoothie

Ingredients

- Espresso: 1 shot (about 30 ml), cooled
- Banana: 1 medium, ripe
- Almond milk: 1 cup (unsweetened)
- Cocoa powder: 1 tablespoon
- Ice cubes: a handful (optional)

Nutritional Info

- Calories: 150-200 kcal
- Protein: 3-4 g
- Carbohydrates: 30-35 g
- Dietary fiber: 4-5 g
- Sugars: 15-20 g
- Fat: 2-3 g
- Saturated Fat: 0 g
- Cholesterol: 0 mg
- Sodium: 100-150 mg
- Potassium: 500-550 mg
- Vitamin C: 10 mg
- Calcium: 300-350 mg
- Iron: 1 mg

⏲ Preparation Time: 05m

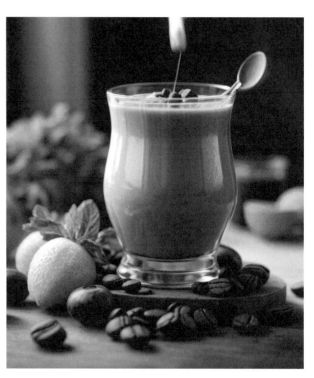

Directions

- Prepare the Ingredients: Brew a shot of espresso and let it cool. Peel the banana.
- Blending: In a blender, combine the cooled espresso, banana, almond milk, and cocoa powder. Add ice cubes if you prefer a chilled smoothie.
- Blending Speed and Time: Blend on high speed for about 60 seconds, or until the smoothie is smooth and creamy.
- Taste and Adjust: If the smoothie is too thick, add a bit more almond milk. Adjust sweetness if necessary, perhaps with a teaspoon of honey or agave syrup.
- Serve Immediately: Pour into a glass and enjoy your energizing Espresso Energy Booster smoothie!

Tips and Techniques

- Ingredient Alternatives: If you don't have espresso, you can use strong brewed coffee instead. If almond milk is not available, any plant-based milk like soy or oat milk can be used.
- Nutrition Boost: For added protein, include a scoop of your favorite protein powder. You can also add a tablespoon of chia seeds for extra fiber and omega-3 fatty acids.
- Storage: Best consumed immediately for maximum freshness and flavor.
- The Espresso Energy Booster smoothie is a perfect combination of coffee and nutrition, making it an excellent choice for a morning drink to wake up and energize your day!

Sunrise Citrus Burst Smoothie

Ingredients

Preparation Time: 05m

- Orange: 1 large, peeled and segmented
- Carrot: 1 medium, peeled and chopped
- Fresh ginger: 1 small piece (about 1/2 inch), peeled and grated
- Pineapple juice: 1/2 cup (fresh or unsweetened)

Nutritional Info

- Calories: 120-150 kcal
- Protein: 2-3 g
- Carbohydrates: 30-35 g
- Dietary fiber: 4-5 g
- Sugars: 20-25 g
- Fat: 0.5 g
- Saturated Fat: 0 g
- Cholesterol: 0 mg
- Sodium: 40-60 mg
- Potassium: 400-500 mg
- Vitamin A: 10,000 IU
- Vitamin C: 80-100 mg
- Calcium: 50-70 mg
- Iron: 0.5 mg

Directions

- Prepare the Ingredients: Peel and segment the orange, ensuring to remove any seeds. Peel and chop the carrot. Peel and grate the ginger.
- Blending: In a blender, combine the orange segments, chopped carrot, grated ginger, and pineapple juice.
- Blending Speed and Time: Blend on high speed for about 60 seconds, or until the smoothie is smooth and the ingredients are fully integrated.
- Taste and Adjust: If the smoothie is too thick, add a bit more pineapple juice or water. Adjust sweetness if necessary, perhaps with a teaspoon of honey or agave syrup.
- Serve Immediately: Pour into glasses and enjoy your refreshing Sunrise Citrus Burst smoothie!

Tips and Techniques

- Ingredient Alternatives: If pineapple juice is not available, you can use apple juice or a mix of orange and lemon juice.
- Nutrition Boost: Add a tablespoon of chia seeds or ground flaxseed for added fiber and omega-3 fatty acids.
- Storage: Best consumed immediately for maximum freshness and nutrient retention. However, if needed, it can be stored in the refrigerator for up to 24 hours. Stir well before drinking.
- The Sunrise Citrus Burst smoothie is a delightful way to kick off your morning with a blend of fresh, zesty flavors and a nutritious boost!

Avocado Green Kick Smoothie

Ingredients

- Avocado: 1/2 medium, pitted and scooped
- Spinach: 1 cup, fresh
- Apple juice: 1 cup (preferably fresh or unsweetened)
- Lemon juice: from 1/2 lemon

Nutritional Info

- Calories: 250-300 kcal
- Protein: 3-4 g
- Carbohydrates: 30-35 g
- Dietary Fiber: 7-8 g
- Sugars: 15-20 g
- Fat: 15-18 g
- Saturated Fat: 2-3 g
- Cholesterol: 0 mg
- Sodium: 30-50 mg
- Potassium: 800-900 mg
- Vitamin A: 2900 IU
- Vitamin C: 40-50 mg
- Calcium: 50-70 mg
- Iron: 1.5 mg

Directions

- Prepare the Ingredients: Halve the avocado, remove the pit, and scoop out the flesh. Wash the spinach leaves. Squeeze the lemon for juice.
- Blending: In a blender, combine the avocado, spinach, apple juice, and lemon juice.
- Blending Speed and Time: Blend on high speed for about 60 seconds, or until the smoothie is smooth and creamy.
- Taste and Adjust: If the smoothie is too thick, add a bit more apple juice. Adjust sweetness or tartness as needed, perhaps with a bit more lemon juice or a teaspoon of honey.
- Serve Immediately: Pour into glasses and enjoy your nourishing Avocado Green Kick smoothie!

Tips and Techniques

- Ingredient Alternatives: If apple juice is not available, you can use any other fruit juice like pear or orange juice. For added protein, include a scoop of your favorite protein powder.
- Nutrition Boost: Add a tablespoon of chia seeds or ground flaxseed for extra fiber and omega-3 fatty acids.
- Storage: Best consumed immediately. However, if necessary, it can be stored in the refrigerator for up to 24 hours. Stir well before drinking.
- The Avocado Green Kick smoothie is a fantastic choice for a morning drink, offering a delicious blend of flavors and a boost of energy and nutrients!

Simple Seasonal Smoothies

Green Apple Energizer Smoothie

Ingredients

- Green apples: 1 large, cored and chopped
- Spinach: 1 cup, fresh
- Honey: 1 tablespoon (adjust to taste)
- Coconut milk: 1 cup
- Ice cubes: a handful (optional)

Nutritional Info

- Calories: 200-250 kcal
- Protein: 2-3 g
- Carbohydrates: 35-40 g
- Dietary fiber: 4-5 g
- Sugars: 25-30 g
- Fat: 8-10 g
- Sodium: 50-70 mg
- Potassium: 400-500 mg
- Vitamin A: 2900 IU
- Vitamin C: 15-20 mg
- Calcium: 40-50 mg
- Iron: 1.5 mg

Directions

- Wash, core, and chop the green apple. Rinse the spinach leaves. In a blender, combine the chopped green apple, spinach, honey, and coconut milk. Add ice cubes if you prefer a colder smoothie.
- Blend on high speed for about 60 seconds, until the smoothie is creamy. If the smoothie is too thick, add a bit more milk. Adjust sweetness with additional honey. Pour into glasses and enjoy a smoothie!

Tips and Techniques

- If you don't have coconut milk, you can use almond milk or another plant-based milk. For an extra protein boost, add a scoop of your favorite protein powder.
- Add a tablespoon of chia seeds or ground flaxseed for added fiber and omega-3 fatty acids.
- Best consumed immediately. However, if necessary, it can be stored in the refrigerator for up to 24 hours. Stir well before drinking.

Pineapple Ginger Revive Smoothie

Ingredients

- Pineapple: 1 cup, chopped (fresh or frozen)
- Fresh ginger: 1-inch piece, peeled and grated
- Banana: 1 medium, ripe
- Greek yogurt: 1/2 cup (non-fat or low-fat)
- Ice cubes: a handful (optional)
- Honey or agave syrup: 1 tablespoon (optional)

Nutritional Info

- Calories: 200-250 kcal
- Protein: 6-8 g
- Carbohydrates: 45-50 g
- Dietary Fiber: 3-4 g
- Sugars: 30-35 g
- Fat: 0.5-1 g
- Cholesterol: 5 mg
- Sodium: 50-70 mg
- Potassium: 500-600 mg
- Vitamin C: 50-60 mg
- Calcium: 150-200 mg
- Iron: 0.5 mg

Directions

- Chop the pineapple if using fresh. Peel and grate the ginger. Peel the banana. In a blender, combine the pineapple, grated ginger, banana, Greek yogurt, and ice cubes.
- Add honey or agave syrup if you prefer a sweeter smoothie. Blend on high speed for about 60 seconds, or until the smoothie is smooth and creamy.
- If the smoothie is too thick, add a bit more water or yogurt. Adjust sweetness if necessary with additional honey or agave syrup. Pour into glasses and enjoy your revitalizing smoothie!

Tips and Techniques

- For a vegan option, use a plant-based yogurt and sweetener.
- Add a tablespoon of chia seeds or ground flaxseed for extra fiber and omega-3 fatty acids.
- Best consumed immediately for maximum freshness and flavor. However, it can be stored in the refrigerator for up to 24 hours if needed. Stir well before drinking.

🕐 **Preparation Time:** 05m

Cranberry Citrus Wake-up Smoothie

Ingredients

- Cranberries: 1 cup, fresh or frozen
- Orange juice: 1 cup (freshly squeezed)
- Honey: 1 tablespoon (adjust to taste)
- Greek yogurt: 1/2 cup (non-fat or low-fat)
- Ice cubes: a handful (optional)

Nutritional Info

- Calories: 150-200 kcal
- Protein: 1-2 g
- Carbohydrates: 35-40 g
- Dietary Fiber: 3-4 g
- Sugars: 30-35 g
- Fat: 0.5 g
- Cholesterol: 0 mg
- Sodium: 10-20 mg
- Potassium: 300-400 mg
- Vitamin C: 60-70 mg
- Calcium: 20-30 mg
- Iron: 0.5 mg

Directions

- If using fresh cranberries, wash them thoroughly.
- In a blender, combine the cranberries, orange juice, honey, and Greek yogurt (if using). Add ice cubes for a chilled smoothie
- Blend on high speed for about 60 seconds, or until the smoothie is smooth and the cranberries are fully blended.
- If the smoothie is too tart, add more honey. If it's too thick, add a bit more orange juice.
- Pour into glasses and enjoy your vibrant and tangy Cranberry Citrus Wake-up smoothie!

Tips and Techniques

- If Greek yogurt is not available or you prefer a dairy-free option, you can omit it or use a plant-based yogurt alternative.
- Add a tablespoon of chia seeds or ground flaxseed for added fiber, omega-3 fatty acids, and nutrients.
- Best consumed immediately for maximum freshness and flavor. However, it can be refrigerated for up to 24 hours if needed. Stir well before drinking.

Strawberry Banana Classic Smoothie

Ingredients

- Strawberries: 1 cup, fresh or frozen
- Banana: 1 medium, ripe
- Greek yogurt: 1/2 cup (plain, non-fat or low-fat)
- Milk: 1/2 cup (cow's, almond, or soy)
- Ice cubes: a handful (optional)
- Honey or agave syrup: 1 tablespoon (optional)

Nutritional Info

- Calories: 200-250 kcal
- Protein: 8-10 g
- Carbohydrates: 40-45 g
- Dietary fiber: 4-5 g
- Sugars: 25-30 g
- Fat: 0.5-1 g
- Saturated Fat: 0 g
- Cholesterol: 5 mg
- Sodium: 50-100 mg
- Potassium: 500-600 mg
- Vitamin C: 60-70 mg
- Calcium: 150-200 mg
- Iron: 0.5 mg

Directions

- Prepare the Ingredients: Wash the strawberries if using fresh. Peel the banana.
- Blending: In a blender, combine the strawberries, banana, Greek yogurt, milk, and ice cubes. Add honey or agave syrup if you prefer a sweeter smoothie.
- Blending Speed and Time: Blend on high speed for about 60 seconds, or until the smoothie is smooth and creamy.
- Taste and Adjust: If the smoothie is too thick, add more milk. If it's not sweet enough, add a bit more honey or agave syrup.
- Serve Immediately: Pour into glasses and enjoy your classic Strawberry Banana smoothie!

Tips and Techniques

- For a vegan option, replace Greek yogurt with plant-based yogurt and use plant-based milk. You can also add a scoop of protein powder for an extra protein boost.
- Add a tablespoon of chia seeds or ground flaxseed for added fiber and omega-3 fatty acids.
- This smoothie is best enjoyed fresh. However, if necessary, it can be stored in the refrigerator for up to 24 hours. Stir well before drinking.

Berry Melon Refresh Smoothie

Ingredients

- Watermelon: 2 cups, cubed and seedless
- Raspberries: 1 cup, fresh or frozen
- Lemon juice: from 1 medium lemon
- Ice cubes: a handful (optional, recommended if using fresh raspberries)
- Honey or agave syrup: 1 tablespoon (optional)

Nutritional Info

- Calories: 100-150 kcal
- Protein: 2-3 g
- Carbohydrates: 25-30 g
- Dietary Fiber: 3-4 g
- Sugars: 20-25 g
- Fat: 0.5 g
- Cholesterol: 0 mg
- Sodium: 10-20 mg
- Potassium: 300-400 mg
- Vitamin C: 40-50 mg
- Calcium: 20-30 mg
- Iron: 0.5 mg

Directions

- Cube the watermelon and ensure it's seedless. Wash the raspberries if using fresh. Squeeze the lemon for juice.
- In a blender, combine the watermelon, raspberries, lemon juice, and ice cubes. Add honey or agave syrup if you prefer a sweeter smoothie.
- Blend on high speed for about 60 seconds, or until the smoothie is smooth and well-mixed.
- Taste and Adjust: If the smoothie is too thick, add a little water. If it's not sweet enough, add a bit more honey or agave syrup.
- Pour into glasses and enjoy your refreshing Berry Melon Refresh smoothie!

Tips and Techniques

- If raspberries are not available, you can use strawberries or blueberries for a similar berry flavor.
- Add a tablespoon of chia seeds or ground flaxseed for added fiber and omega-3 fatty acids.
- Best consumed immediately, especially since watermelon's texture can change when stored. However, if necessary, it can be refrigerated for a few hours. Stir well before drinking.

🕐 **Preparation Time:** 05m

Mango Madness Smoothie

Ingredients

- Ripe mangoes: 2 cups, peeled and cubed
- Lime juice: from 1 medium lime
- Greek yogurt: 1/2 cup (plain, non-fat)
- Honey or agave syrup: 1 tablespoon
- Ice cubes: a handful (optional)
- Water or coconut water: 1/2 cup

Nutritional Info

- Calories: 150-200 kcal
- Protein: 2-3 g
- Carbohydrates: 35-40 g
- Dietary Fiber: 3-4 g
- Sugars: 30-35 g
- Fat: 0.5 g
- Cholesterol: 0 mg
- Sodium: 10-20 mg
- Potassium: 500-600 mg
- Vitamin C: 60-70 mg
- Calcium: 20-30 mg
- Iron: 0.5 mg

Directions

- Peel and cube the mangoes. Squeeze the lime for juice.
- In a blender, combine the mango cubes, lime juice, Greek yogurt (if using), honey or agave syrup (if desired), and ice cubes. Add water or coconut water to adjust the consistency.
- Blend on high speed for about 60 seconds, or until the smoothie is smooth and creamy.
- If the smoothie is too thick, add more water or coconut water. Adjust sweetness if necessary with more honey or agave syrup. Pour into glasses and enjoy your delicious Mango Madness smoothie!

Tips and Techniques

- If Greek yogurt is not available or if you prefer a dairy-free option, you can omit it or use a plant-based yogurt.
- Add a tablespoon of chia seeds or ground flaxseed for added fiber and omega-3 fatty acids.
- This smoothie is best enjoyed fresh. However, if necessary, it can be stored in the refrigerator for up to 24 hours. Stir well before drinking.

Cherry Vanilla Dream Smoothie

Ingredients

- Sweet cherries: 1 cup, pitted (fresh or frozen)
- Vanilla almond milk: 1 cup (unsweetened)
- Greek yogurt: 1/2 cup (plain, non-fat or low-fat)
- Vanilla extract: 1/2 teaspoon (for almond milk)
- Honey or agave syrup: 1 tablespoon (optional)
- Ice cubes: a handful (optional)

Nutritional Info

- Calories: 150-200 kcal
- Protein: 2-3 g
- Carbohydrates: 30-35 g
- Dietary Fiber: 3-4 g
- Sugars: 25-30 g
- Fat: 2-3 g
- Cholesterol: 0 mg
- Sodium: 100-150 mg
- Potassium: 300-400 mg
- Vitamin C: 10-15 mg
- Calcium: 300-350 mg
- Iron: 1 mg

Directions

- If using fresh cherries, wash and pit them. If using frozen cherries, they're ready to use.
- In a blender, combine the cherries, vanilla almond milk, Greek yogurt (if using), vanilla extract (if needed), and honey or agave syrup. Add ice cubes for a colder smoothie.
- Blend on high speed for about 60 seconds, or until the smoothie is smooth and creamy.
- If the smoothie is too thick, add more almond milk. Adjust sweetness if necessary with additional honey or agave syrup.
- Pour into glasses and enjoy your Cherry Vanilla Dream smoothie!

Tips and Techniques

- If vanilla almond milk is not available, you can use regular almond milk and increase the vanilla extract. For a dairy-free version, omit the Greek yogurt or use a plant-based yogurt.
- Add a tablespoon of chia seeds or ground flaxseed for extra fiber and omega-3 fatty acids.
- Best consumed immediately. However, if necessary, it can be stored in the refrigerator for up to 24 hours. Stir well before drinking.

Pear Vanilla Harmony Smoothie

Ingredients

- Pear: 1 large, ripe, cored and chopped
- Vanilla yogurt: 1 cup (or Greek yogurt)
- Fresh mint leaves: a handful (about 8-10 leaves)
- Honey or agave syrup: 1 tablespoon (optional)
- Ice cubes: a handful (optional)
- Almond milk or water: 1/2 cup (for desired consistency)

Nutritional Info

- Calories: 200-250 kcal
- Protein: 6-10 g
- Carbohydrates: 40-45 g
- Dietary Fiber: 5-6 g
- Sugars: 30-35 g
- Fat: 2-3 g
- Saturated Fat: 1 g
- Cholesterol: 5 mg
- Sodium: 50-100 mg
- Potassium: 400-500 mg
- Vitamin A: 100 IU
- Vitamin C: 10 mg
- Calcium: 200-250 mg
- Iron: 0.5 mg

Directions

- Wash, core, and chop the pear. Rinse the mint leaves.
- In a blender, combine the chopped pear, vanilla yogurt, fresh mint leaves, and honey or agave syrup. Add ice cubes for a colder smoothie. Add almond milk or water to adjust the consistency.
- Blend on high speed for about 60 seconds, or until the smoothie is smooth and creamy.
- If the smoothie is too thick, add more almond milk or water. Adjust sweetness if necessary with more honey or agave syrup. Pour into glasses and enjoy your Pear Vanilla Harmony smoothie!

Tips and Techniques

- If vanilla yogurt is not available, you can use plain yogurt with a splash of vanilla extract. For a vegan option, use plant-based yogurt and milk.
- Add a tablespoon of chia seeds or ground flaxseed for added fiber and omega-3 fatty acids.
- Best consumed immediately. However, if necessary, it can be stored in the refrigerator for up to 24 hours. Stir well before drinking.

🕒 **Preparation Time:** 05m

Pomegranate Power Punch Smoothie

Ingredients

- Pomegranate juice: 1 cup
- Blueberries: 1 cup, fresh or frozen
- Honey: 1 tablespoon (adjust to taste)
- Greek yogurt: 1/2 cup (non-fat or low-fat)
- Ice cubes: a handful (optional)

Nutritional Info

- Calories: 150-200 kcal
- Protein: 1-2 g
- Carbohydrates: 35-40 g
- Dietary Fiber: 3-4 g
- Sugars: 30-35 g
- Fat: 0.5 g
- Cholesterol: 0 mg
- Sodium: 20-30 mg
- Potassium: 300-400 mg
- Vitamin C: 20-30 mg
- Calcium: 20-30 mg
- Iron: 0.5 mg

Directions

- If using fresh blueberries, wash them thoroughly.
- In a blender, combine the pomegranate juice, blueberries, honey, and Greek yogurt (if using). Add ice cubes for a chilled smoothie.
- Blend on high speed for about 60 seconds, or until the smoothie is smooth and creamy.
- If the smoothie is too thick, add a bit more pomegranate juice. Adjust sweetness if necessary with additional honey. Pour into glasses and enjoy your refreshing Pomegranate Power Punch smoothie!

Tips and Techniques

- If Greek yogurt is not available or if you prefer a dairy-free option, you can omit it or use a plant-based yogurt alternative.
- Add a tablespoon of chia seeds or ground flaxseed for extra fiber and omega-3 fatty acids.
- Best consumed immediately. However, if necessary, it can be refrigerated for up to 24 hours. Stir well before drinking.

CHAPTER 8

Tropical Smoothie Escape

🕐 **Preparation Time:** 10m

Lychee Coconut Dream Smoothie

Ingredients

- Lychees: 1 cup, peeled and pitted (fresh or canned in syrup, drained)
- Coconut milk: 1 cup (or coconut milk)
- Lime juice: from 1/2 lime
- Ice cubes: a handful (optional)
- Honey or agave syrup: 1 tablespoon (optional, adjust to taste)

Nutritional Info

- Calories: 200-250 kcal
- Protein: 2-3 g
- Carbohydrates: 30-35 g
- Dietary Fiber: 2-3 g
- Sugars: 20-25 g
- Fat: 10-12 g
- Saturated Fat: 9-10 g
- Cholesterol: 0 mg
- Sodium: 20-30 mg
- Potassium: 300-350 mg
- Vitamin C: 30-40 mg
- Calcium: 30-40 mg
- Iron: 1-2 mg

Directions

- Prepare the Ingredients: Peel and pit the lychees if using fresh. If using canned lychees, drain them from the syrup.
- Blending: In a blender, combine the lychees, coconut milk, lime juice, and ice cubes. Add honey or agave syrup for extra sweetness, if desired.
- Blending Speed and Time: Blend on high speed for about 60 seconds, or until the smoothie is smooth and creamy.
- Taste and Adjust: If the smoothie is too thick, add a bit more coconut milk. Adjust the sweetness or tartness to your liking. Serve Immediately: Pour into glasses and enjoy your smooth and tropical Lychee Coconut Dream smoothie!

Tips and Techniques

- Ingredient Alternatives: If lychees are not available, you can use rambutan or a similar tropical fruit. If you prefer a dairy-based smoothie, substitute coconut milk with regular milk or a plant-based milk of your choice.
- Nutrition Boost: Add a scoop of your favorite protein powder or a tablespoon of chia seeds for extra nutrients.
- Storage: Best consumed immediately to enjoy the fresh flavors. However, if necessary, it can be refrigerated for a few hours. Stir well before drinking.
- The Lychee Coconut Dream smoothie is a wonderfully exotic and refreshing drink, perfect for adding a touch of the tropics to your smoothie collection!

Dragon Fruit Delight Smoothie

Ingredients

- Dragon fruit (pitaya): 1 large or 2 small, peeled and chopped
- Kiwi: 2, peeled and sliced
- Coconut milk: 1 cup
- Ice cubes: a handful (optional)
- Honey or agave syrup: 1 tablespoon (optional)
- Fresh lime juice: from 1/2 lime (optional)

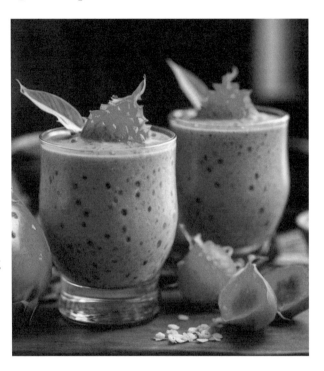

Nutritional Info

- Calories: 200-250 kcal
- Protein: 2-3 g
- Carbohydrates: 40-45 g
- Dietary Fiber: 5-6 g
- Sugars: 25-30 g
- Fat: 5-7 g
- Saturated Fat: 4-5 g
- Cholesterol: 0 mg
- Sodium: 50-70 mg
- Potassium: 500-600 mg
- Vitamin C: 40-50 mg
- Calcium: 40-50 mg
- Iron: 1-2 mg

Directions

- Prepare the Ingredients: Slice the dragon fruit and kiwi. If you're using fresh dragon fruit, you can freeze the chunks beforehand for a colder smoothie.
- Blending: In a blender, combine the dragon fruit, kiwi slices, coconut milk, and ice cubes. Add honey or agave syrup for extra sweetness and lime juice for a citrusy kick, if desired.
- Blending Speed and Time: Blend on high speed for about 60 seconds, or until the smoothie is smooth and creamy.
- Taste and Adjust: If the smoothie is too thick, add a bit more coconut milk. Adjust the sweetness or tartness to your liking.
- Serve Immediately: Pour into glasses and enjoy your vibrant and exotic Dragon Fruit Delight smoothie!

Tips and Techniques

- Ingredient Alternatives: If dragon fruit is not available, you can use frozen dragon fruit puree. If coconut milk is too rich, you can substitute it with almond milk or another plant-based milk.
- Nutrition Boost: Add a scoop of your favorite protein powder or a tablespoon of chia seeds for an extra nutrient kick.
- Storage: This smoothie is best enjoyed fresh to maximize the benefits and flavors of the ingredients. However, it can be refrigerated for a few hours if necessary.
- The Dragon Fruit Delight smoothie is an excellent way to enjoy the unique flavors of tropical fruits in a delicious and healthy drink!

Passion Fruit Paradise Smoothie

Ingredients

- Passion fruit: 2-3 fruits, pulp scooped out
- Pineapple: 1 cup, chopped (fresh or frozen)
- Mango: 1 cup, chopped (fresh or frozen)
- Lemon juice: from 1 medium lemon
- Ice cubes: a handful (optional)
- Honey or agave syrup: 1 tablespoon (optional)
- Water or coconut water: 1/2 cup

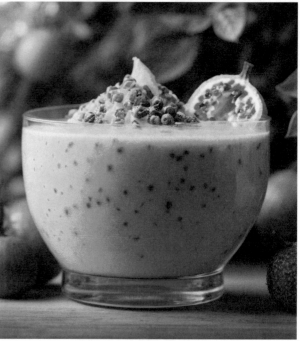

Nutritional Info

- Calories: 200-250 kcal
- Protein: 2-3 g
- Carbohydrates: 50-55 g
- Dietary Fiber: 5-6 g
- Sugars: 40-45 g
- Fat: 1-2 g
- Saturated Fat: 0 g
- Cholesterol: 0 mg
- Sodium: 10-20 mg
- Potassium: 500-600 mg
- Vitamin C: 100-120 mg
- Calcium: 30-40 mg
- Iron: 1-1.5 mg

Directions

- Prepare the Ingredients: Cut the passion fruit in half and scoop out the pulp. Chop the pineapple and mango if using fresh.
- Blending: In a blender, combine the passion fruit pulp, chopped pineapple, mango, lemon juice, and ice cubes. Add honey or agave syrup for extra sweetness, if desired. Add water or coconut water to adjust the consistency.
- Blending Speed and Time: Blend on high speed for about 60 seconds, or until the smoothie is smooth and creamy.
- Taste and Adjust: If the smoothie is too thick, add more water or coconut water. Adjust the sweetness or tartness to your liking. Serve Immediately: Pour into glasses and enjoy your tropical smoothie!

Tips and Techniques

- Ingredient Alternatives: If fresh passion fruit is not available, you can use frozen or canned passion fruit pulp.
- Nutrition Boost: Add a tablespoon of chia seeds or ground flaxseed for extra fiber and omega-3 fatty acids.
- Storage: Best enjoyed fresh. However, if necessary, it can be stored in the refrigerator for a few hours. Stir well before drinking.
- The Passion Fruit Paradise smoothie is an excellent choice for a nutrient-rich and flavor-packed drink, perfect for those who enjoy exotic and tropical tastes!

Tropical Guava Glow Smoothie

Ingredients

🕐 **Preparation Time:** 15m

- Guava: 2 medium-sized, peeled and seeded
- Banana: 1 medium, ripe
- Mint syrup: 1 tablespoon
- Greek yogurt: 1/2 cup (plain, non-fat or low-fat) for added creaminess (optional)
- Ice cubes: a handful (optional)
- Coconut water or regular water: 1/2 cup

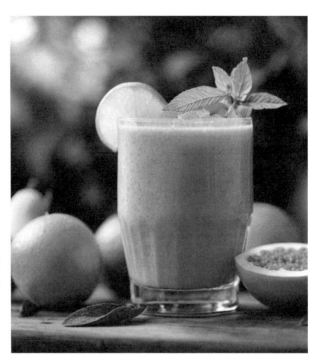

Nutritional Info

- Calories: 180-230 kcal
- Protein: 2-4 g
- Carbohydrates: 40-45 g
- Dietary Fiber: 5-6 g
- Sugars: 30-35 g
- Fat: 1-2 g
- Saturated Fat: 0.5 g
- Cholesterol: 0 mg
- Sodium: 20-30 mg
- Potassium: 500-600 mg
- Vitamin C: 200-250 mg
- Calcium: 30-40 mg
- Iron: 0.5-1 mg

Directions

- Prepare the Ingredients: Peel and seed the guavas. Peel the banana.
- Blending: In a blender, combine the guavas, banana, mint syrup, Greek yogurt (if using), and ice cubes. Add coconut water or regular water to adjust the consistency.
- Blending Speed and Time: Blend on high speed for about 60 seconds, or until the smoothie is smooth and creamy.
- Taste and Adjust: If the smoothie is too thick, add more coconut water or regular water. Adjust the sweetness or mint flavor to your liking.
- Serve Immediately: Pour into glasses and enjoy your aromatic and refreshing Tropical Guava Glow smoothie!

Tips and Techniques

- Ingredient Alternatives: If guava is not available, you can use guava juice or nectar. If you prefer a vegan option, omit the Greek yogurt or use a plant-based yogurt.
- Nutrition Boost: For added nutrients, include a tablespoon of chia seeds or ground flaxseeds.
- Storage: Best consumed immediately. However, if necessary, it can be stored in the refrigerator for up to 24 hours. Stir well before drinking.
- The Tropical Guava Glow smoothie is a delightful and nutritious drink, perfect for bringing a taste of the tropics to your day!

Mango Papaya Samba Smoothie

Ingredients

- Mango: 1 cup, peeled and chopped (fresh or frozen)
- Papaya: 1 cup, peeled, seeded, and chopped
- Orange juice: 1/2 cup (freshly squeezed)
- Greek yogurt: 1/2 cup (non-fat or low-fat)
- Ice cubes: a handful (optional)
- Honey or agave syrup: 1 tablespoon (optional)

Nutritional Info

- Calories: 200-250 kcal
- Protein: 2-4 g
- Carbohydrates: 50-55 g
- Dietary fiber: 4-5 g
- Sugars: 40-45 g
- Fat: 1-2 g
- Saturated Fat: 0.5 g
- Cholesterol: 0 mg
- Sodium: 20-30 mg
- Potassium: 600-700 mg
- Vitamin C: 150-200 mg
- Calcium: 30-40 mg
- Iron: 1 mg

Directions

- Prepare the Ingredients: Peel and chop the mango and papaya.
- Blending: In a blender, combine the mango, papaya, orange juice, Greek yogurt (if using), and ice cubes. Add honey or agave syrup for extra sweetness, if desired.
- Blending Speed and Time: Blend on high speed for about 60 seconds, or until the smoothie is smooth and creamy.
- Taste and Adjust: If the smoothie is too thick, add a bit more orange juice. Adjust the sweetness to your liking.
- Serve Immediately: Pour into glasses and enjoy your tropical Mango Papaya Samba smoothie!

Tips and Techniques

- Ingredient Alternatives: If Greek yogurt is not available or if you prefer a vegan option, you can omit it or use a plant-based yogurt alternative.
- Nutrition Boost: For added nutrients, include a scoop of protein powder or a tablespoon of chia seeds or ground flaxseed.
- Storage: Best consumed immediately. However, if necessary, it can be refrigerated for up to 24 hours. Stir well before drinking.
- The Mango Papaya Samba smoothie is a delightful way to enjoy the exotic flavors of the tropics in a delicious and healthy drink!

CHAPTER 9

Diabetic-Friendly Smoothies

○ **Preparation Time:** 10m

Turmeric Sunrise Soothing Smoothie

Ingredients

- Carrot: 1 medium, peeled and chopped
- Unsweetened coconut water: 1 cup
- Ground turmeric: 1/2 teaspoon
- Fresh ginger: 1/2-inch piece, grated
- Lemon juice: from 1/2 lemon
- Cinnamon: 1/2 teaspoon

Nutritional Info

- Calories: 80-120 kcal
- Protein: 1-2 g
- Carbohydrates: 15-20 g
- Dietary Fiber: 3-4 g
- Sugars: 6-8 g
- Fat: 0.5 g
- Cholesterol: 0 mg
- Sodium: 50-100 mg
- Potassium: 400-500 mg
- Vitamin C: 15-20 mg
- Calcium: 40-50 mg
- Iron: 0.5 mg

Directions

- Chop the carrot. Grate the fresh turmeric and ginger. In a blender, combine the chopped carrot, coconut water, grated turmeric, grated ginger, lemon juice, cinnamon, ice cubes, and stevia or sweetener if using.
- Blend on high speed for about 60 seconds, or until the smoothie is smooth and the ingredients are well incorporated.
- Adjust the sweetness with more stevia or sweetener, if needed. Add more coconut water if the smoothie is too thick. Pour into glasses and enjoy your refreshing Turmeric Sunrise Soother smoothie!

Tips and Techniques

- If fresh turmeric isn't available, ground turmeric can be used. You can also add a small amount of orange or apple for additional sweetness, but be mindful of the sugar content.
- Add a tablespoon of chia seeds or flaxseeds for extra fiber and omega-3 fatty acids.
- Best consumed immediately. If needed, it can be stored in the refrigerator for up to 24 hours. Stir well before drinking.

Green Glycemic Guardian Smoothie

Ingredients

- Spinach: 1 cup, fresh
- Kale: 1/2 cup, fresh, stems removed
- Cucumber: 1/2 medium, peeled and sliced
- Green apple: 1/2, cored and chopped (optional)
- Avocado: 1/4, peeled and pitted for creaminess
- Lemon juice: from 1/2 lemon
- Fresh ginger: 1-inch piece, peeled and grated
- Chia seeds: 1 tablespoon
- Unsweetened almond milk or water: 1 cup
- Ice cubes: a handful (optional)

Directions

- Wash the spinach, kale, cucumber, and green apple. Peel and chop the ginger.
- In a blender, combine spinach, kale, cucumber, green apple (if using), avocado, lemon juice, grated ginger, chia seeds, and almond milk or water. Add ice cubes if you prefer a colder smoothie.
- Blend on high speed for about 60 seconds, or until the smoothie is smooth and creamy.
- Adjust the consistency by adding more almond milk or water if needed. You can also add a natural sweetener like stevia if desired.
- Pour into glasses and enjoy your nutrient-rich Green Glycemic Guardian smoothie!

Nutritional Info

- Calories: 150-200 kcal
- Protein: 3-5 g
- Carbohydrates: 15-20 g
- Dietary Fiber: 6-8 g
- Sugars: 4-6 g
- Fat: 8-10 g
- Saturated Fat: 1-1.5 g
- Sodium: 50-100 mg
- Potassium: 500-600 mg
- Vitamin C: 60-80 mg
- Calcium: 150-200 mg
- Iron: 2-3 mg

Tips and Techniques

- If you prefer, you can replace kale with additional spinach or another leafy green like Swiss chard.
- Best consumed immediately for maximum freshness. However, it can be stored in the refrigerator for up to 24 hours. Stir well before drinking.

Berry Balanced Boost Smoothie

Ingredients

- Mixed berries: 1 cup, fresh or frozen
- Unsweetened almond milk: 1 cup
- Chia seeds: 1 tablespoon
- Greek yogurt: 1/2 cup (non-fat or low-fat)
- Low-calorie sweetener: to taste
- Ice cubes: a handful (optional)

Nutritional Info

- Calories: 120-150 kcal
- Protein: 2-4 g
- Carbohydrates: 20-25 g
- Dietary Fiber: 6-8 g
- Sugars: 10-12 g
- Fat: 4-5 g
- Saturated Fat: 0.5 g
- Sodium: 50-70 mg
- Potassium: 200-300 mg
- Vitamin C: 30-50 mg
- Calcium: 150-200 mg
- Iron: 1 mg

Directions

- If using fresh berries, wash them thoroughly. In a blender, combine the mixed berries, almond milk, chia seeds, Greek yogurt (if using), and stevia or sweetener (if desired). Add ice cubes for a chilled smoothie.
- Blend on high speed for about 60 seconds, or until the smoothie is smooth and creamy.
- If the smoothie is too thick, add more almond milk. Adjust the sweetness to your liking with additional stevia or sweetener. Pour into glasses and enjoy your Berry Balanced Boost smoothie!

Tips and Techniques

- You can use any combination of low-glycemic berries available to you. For a dairy-free version, omit the Greek yogurt or use a plant-based yogurt.
- Add a scoop of unsweetened protein powder for an extra protein kick. Best consumed immediately for maximum freshness. However, it can be stored in the refrigerator for up to 24 hours. Stir well before drinking.

🕐 **Preparation Time:** 10m

Cinnamon Spice Stabilizer Smoothie

Ingredients

- Unsweetened almond milk: 1 cup
- Ground cinnamon: 1 teaspoon
- Small apple: 1, cored and chopped
- Ground flaxseeds: 1 tablespoon
- Greek yogurt: 1/2 cup (non-fat or low-fat)
- Vanilla extract: 1/2 teaspoon
- Low-calorie sweetener: to taste

Nutritional Info

- Calories: 100-150 kcal
- Protein: 2-3 g
- Carbohydrates: 15-20 g
- Dietary fiber: 4-5 g
- Sugars: 10-12 g
- Fat: 3-4 g
- Saturated Fat: 0 g
- Cholesterol: 0 mg
- Sodium: 50-70 mg
- Potassium: 200-250 mg
- Vitamin C: 4-6 mg
- Calcium: 150-200 mg
- Iron: 0.5 mg

Directions

- Wash and chop the apple. In a blender, combine the almond milk, ground cinnamon, chopped apple, ground flaxseeds, Greek yogurt (if using), vanilla extract, and ice cubes. Add stevia or sweetener (if desired) for extra sweetness.
- Blend on high speed for about 60 seconds, or until the smoothie is smooth and creamy.
- If the smoothie is too thick, add more almond milk. Adjust the sweetness and spice to your liking. Pour into glasses and enjoy your Cinnamon Spice Stabilizer smoothie!

Tips and Techniques

- For a dairy-free version, omit the Greek yogurt or use a plant-based yogurt. You can also add a scoop of protein powder for extra nutrition.
- Add a handful of spinach or kale for extra vitamins and minerals without significantly impacting the flavor. Best consumed immediately. However, if necessary, it can be stored in the refrigerator for up to 24 hours. Stir well before drinking.

Avocado Almond Bliss Smoothie

Ingredients

- Avocado: 1/2, ripe, pitted and scooped
- Unsweetened almond milk: 1 cup
- Spinach: 1 cup, fresh
- Ground flaxseeds or chia seeds: 1 tablespoon
- Unsweetened protein powder: 1 scoop
- Vanilla extract: 1/2 teaspoon
- Cinnamon: 1/2 teaspoon
- Ice cubes: a handful (optional)
- Low-calorie sweetener: to taste (optional)

Nutritional Info

- Calories: 200-250 kcal
- Protein: 3-5 g
- Carbohydrates: 12-15 g
- Dietary Fiber: 7-8 g
- Sugars: 1-2 g
- Fat: 15-17 g
- Saturated Fat: 2-3 g
- Sodium: 50-100 mg
- Potassium: 500-550 mg
- Vitamin C: 10-15 mg
- Calcium: 300-350 mg
- Iron: 1.5-2 mg

Directions

- Halve the avocado and remove the pit. Scoop out the flesh. Wash the spinach leaves.
- In a blender, combine the avocado, almond milk, spinach, ground flaxseeds or chia seeds, protein powder (if using), vanilla extract, cinnamon, and ice cubes. Add stevia or sweetener (if desired) for extra sweetness.
- Blend on high speed for about 60 seconds, or until the smoothie is smooth and creamy.
- If the smoothie is too thick, add more almond milk. Adjust sweetness and flavor to your liking.
- Pour into glasses and enjoy your nutritious and satisfying Avocado Almond Bliss smoothie!

Tips and Techniques

- You can add a small handful of nuts like almonds or walnuts for extra texture and nutrients.
- For an additional health boost, consider adding a teaspoon of matcha powder or spirulina.
- Best consumed immediately. However, it can be stored in the refrigerator for up to 24 hours. Stir well before drinking.

CHAPTER 10

Smoothie Bowl Creation Bliss

🕐 **Preparation Time:** 05m

Acai Berry Bowl Smoothie

Ingredients

- Acai berry puree: 2 packets (frozen)
- Mixed berries: 1 cup, fresh or frozen
- Banana: 1, ripe, peeled and chopped
- Unsweetened almond milk: 1 cup
- Honey: 1 tablespoon (or to taste) for garnish
- Fresh berries (for garnish): 1/2 cup
- Granola: 1/4 cup for garnish (optional)

Nutritional Info

- Calories: 250-300 kcal
- Protein: 3-5 g
- Carbohydrates: 50-55 g
- Dietary Fiber: 7-9 g
- Sugars: 30-35 g
- Fat: 5-7 g
- Saturated Fat: 1-1.5 g
- Sodium: 50-70 mg
- Potassium: 400-500 mg
- Vitamin C: 30-40 mg
- Calcium: 150-200 mg
- Iron: 1-2 mg

Directions

- Chop the banana and set aside some fresh berries for garnish.
- In a blender, combine the acai berry puree, mixed berries, banana, and almond milk. Add ice cubes for a thicker consistency. Blend on high speed for about 60 seconds, or until the mixture is smooth and creamy. If the mixture is too thick, add a bit more almond milk. Adjust sweetness as needed.
- Pour the smoothie into a bowl. Garnish with fresh berries, a drizzle of honey, and optionally, granola. Serve immediately and relish the flavors of the Acai Berry Bowl!

Tips and Techniques

- If acai puree is not available, acai powder mixed with extra berries can be used. You can also substitute almond milk with another plant-based milk.
- Add a tablespoon of chia seeds or ground flaxseeds for added fiber and omega-3s.

🕐 **Preparation Time:** 10m

Berry Antioxidant Boost Bowl Smoothie

Ingredients

- Blueberries: 1 cup, fresh or frozen
- Raspberries: 1/2 cup, fresh or frozen
- Greek yogurt: 1 cup (plain, non-fat or low-fat)
- Honey: 1 tablespoon (or to taste)
- Fresh berries & coconut flakes for garnish
- Almond milk or water: 1/2 cup

Nutritional Info

- Calories: 200-250 kcal
- Protein: 10-15 g
- Carbohydrates: 35-40 g
- Dietary Fiber: 6-8 g
- Sugars: 25-30 g
- Fat: 2-3 g
- Cholesterol: 5 mg
- Sodium: 50-70 mg
- Potassium: 300-400 mg
- Vitamin C: 20-30 mg
- Calcium: 150-200 mg
- Iron: 1 mg

Directions

- Wash the fresh berries. In a blender, combine blueberries, raspberries, Greek yogurt, honey, and ice cubes. Add almond milk or water to achieve the desired consistency. Blend on high speed for about 60 seconds, or until creamy texture.
- Adjust the sweetness by adding more honey. If the mixture is too thick, add a little more almond milk or water. Pour the smoothie mixture into a bowl. Garnish with fresh berries and coconut flakes.

Tips and Techniques

- You can use any combination of your favorite berries. For a dairy-free version, use plant-based yogurt and sweeteners.
- Add a tablespoon of chia seeds or ground flaxseeds for added fiber and omega-3 fatty acids.
- This smoothie bowl is best enjoyed fresh due to the nature of the ingredients and their textures.

🕐 **Preparation Time:** 10m

Choco Banana Delight Bowl Smoothie

Ingredients

- Bananas: 2 medium-sized, ripe
- Unsweetened cocoa powder: 2 tablespoons
- Unsweetened almond milk: 1 cup
- Ice cubes: a handful (optional)
- Dark chocolate: chopped for garnish
- Honey syrup: 1 tablespoon (optional)
- Granola: 1/4 cup for garnish (optional)

Nutritional Info

- Calories: 300-350 kcal
- Protein: 5-7 g
- Carbohydrates: 50-55 g
- Dietary fiber: 8-10 g
- Sugars: 25-30 g
- Fat: 10-12 g
- Saturated Fat: 5-6 g
- Cholesterol: 0 mg
- Sodium: 50-100 mg
- Potassium: 600-700 mg
- Vitamin C: 10-15 mg
- Calcium: 150-200 mg
- Iron: 2-3 mg

Directions

- Peel and chop one banana for the smoothie. Chop the dark chocolate and slice the second banana for garnish.
- In a blender, combine one chopped banana, unsweetened cocoa powder, almond milk, and ice cubes. Add honey or agave syrup if you prefer a sweeter taste. Blend on high speed for about 60 seconds, or until the mixture is smooth and creamy. If the smoothie is too thick, add a bit more almond milk. Adjust the sweetness as needed.
- Pour the smoothie into a bowl. Garnish with banana slices, dark chocolate chunks, and optionally, granola. Serve immediately and indulge in the rich and satisfying Choco Banana Delight Bowl!

Tips and Techniques

- For a vegan version, ensure that the dark chocolate is dairy-free. You can also add a scoop of protein powder for an extra protein boost.
- Sprinkle with chia seeds or flaxseeds for additional fiber and omega-3 fatty acids.
- This smoothie bowl is best enjoyed fresh due to the fresh ingredients used.

Mango Lassi Bowl Smoothie

Ingredients

- Mango: 1 large, ripe, peeled and chopped (fresh or frozen)
- Greek yogurt: 1 cup
- Honey: 1 tablespoon (adjust to taste)
- Ice cubes: a handful (optional)
- Almond flakes: 1 tablespoon for garnish
- Coconut shavings: 1 tablespoon for garnish

Nutritional Info

- Calories: 250-300 kcal
- Protein: 5-10 g
- Carbohydrates: 45-50 g
- Dietary Fiber: 3-4 g
- Sugars: 35-40 g
- Fat: 5-7 g
- Saturated Fat: 2-3 g
- Cholesterol: 10 mg
- Sodium: 50-100 mg
- Potassium: 400-500 mg
- Vitamin C: 50-60 mg
- Calcium: 150-200 mg
- Iron: 0.5-1 mg

Directions

- Chop the mango and set aside a few small pieces for garnish if desired.
- In a blender, combine the mango, yogurt, and honey. Add ice cubes for a chilled and thicker texture. Blend on high speed for about 60 seconds, or until the mixture is smooth and creamy.
- If the mixture is too thick, add a little more yogurt or a splash of milk. Adjust the sweetness by adding more honey if needed.
- Pour the smoothie into a bowl. Garnish with almond flakes, coconut shavings, and additional mango pieces if you save any.
- Serve immediately and savor the rich and creamy flavors of the Mango Lassi Bowl!

Tips and Techniques

- For a vegan version, use plant-based yogurt and a vegan sweetener like maple syrup.
- You can add a scoop of protein powder or a tablespoon of chia seeds for added nutrients.
- This smoothie bowl is best enjoyed fresh due to the fresh ingredients used.
- This smoothie is a perfect fusion of traditional Indian flavors and the modern trend of smoothie bowls.

Matcha Green Tea Bowl Smoothie

Ingredients

- Matcha green tea powder: 1-2 teaspoons
- Banana: 1 large, ripe, peeled and chopped
- Spinach: 1 cup, fresh
- Unsweetened almond milk: 1 cup
- Mixed fruits: for garnish
- Hemp seeds: 1 tablespoon for garnish
- Honey or agave syrup: 1 tablespoon (optional)

Nutritional Info

- Calories: 200-250 kcal
- Protein: 4-6 g
- Carbohydrates: 35-40 g
- Dietary Fiber: 5-6 g
- Sugars: 15-20 g
- Fat: 5-7 g
- Saturated Fat: 0.5-1 g
- Cholesterol: 0 mg
- Sodium: 50-100 mg
- Potassium: 500-600 mg
- Vitamin C: 20-30 mg
- Calcium: 150-200 mg
- Iron: 2-3 mg

Directions

- Chop the banana and prepare the mixed fruits for garnish.
- In a blender, combine the matcha green tea powder, banana, spinach, and almond milk. Add ice cubes for a thicker texture. Blend on high speed for about 60 seconds, or until the mixture is smooth and creamy. If the smoothie is too thick, add more almond milk. Adjust the sweetness with honey or agave syrup if needed.
- Pour the smoothie into a bowl. Garnish with mixed fruits and sprinkle with hemp seeds. Serve immediately and savor the unique and invigorating Matcha Green Tea Bowl!

Tips and Techniques

- If almond milk is not available, you can use any plant-based milk of your choice. For an extra protein boost, consider adding a scoop of your favorite protein powder.
- You can also add a tablespoon of chia seeds or flaxseeds for added fiber and omega-3 fatty acids. Best consumed immediately. If necessary, it can be refrigerated for a short time before serving.

🕐 **Preparation Time:** 10m

Pumpkin Spice Bowl Smoothie

Ingredients

- Pumpkin puree: 1/2 cup
- Banana: 1 large, ripe, peeled and chopped
- Ground cinnamon: 1 teaspoon
- Nutmeg: 1/4 teaspoon (optional)
- Unsweetened almond milk: 1 cup
- Granola: 1/4 cup for garnish
- Pumpkin seeds: 1 tablespoon for garnish
- Honey syrup: 1 tablespoon (optional)

Nutritional Info

- Calories: 250-300 kcal
- Protein: 4-6 g
- Carbohydrates: 40-45 g
- Dietary Fiber: 6-7 g
- Sugars: 20-25 g
- Fat: 7-9 g
- Saturated Fat: 1-1.5 g
- Cholesterol: 0 mg
- Sodium: 50-100 mg
- Potassium: 500-600 mg
- Vitamin C: 5-10 mg
- Calcium: 150-200 mg
- Iron: 2-3 mg

Directions

- Chop the banana and gather your spices. In a blender, combine the pumpkin puree, banana, ground cinnamon, nutmeg, and almond milk. Add ice cubes for a cooler and thicker consistency. Blend on high speed for about 60 seconds, or until the mixture is smooth and creamy.
- Adjust the sweetness with honey or maple syrup if desired. Add a bit more almond milk if the smoothie is too thick. Pour the smoothie into a bowl. Garnish with granola and pumpkin seeds. Serve immediately and relish the warm and comforting flavors of the Pumpkin Spice Bowl!

Tips and Techniques

- For a vegan version, ensure your granola is vegan-friendly and use maple syrup as a sweetener. You can also add a scoop of protein powder for extra nutrition.
- Sprinkle with chia seeds or flaxseeds for added fiber and omega-3 fatty acids. Best consumed immediately. If necessary, it can be refrigerated for a short time before serving.

Conclusion

As we bring "Smoothie Sensations" to a close, I hope this journey through the vibrant world of smoothies has been as enriching for you as it has been for me. From mastering the basics to exploring advanced creations, this book aims to unlock the endless possibilities that smoothies offer, blending health, flavor, and creativity into every sip.

Smoothies are more than just a drink; they are a lifestyle choice promoting wellness, convenience, and culinary exploration. Whether you're seeking a quick nutritious breakfast, a post-workout recharge, or a delightful dessert alternative, the versatility of smoothies caters to all.

Remember, the art of smoothie-making is an ever-evolving process. I encourage you to keep experimenting with flavors, textures, and ingredients. Your perfect smoothie is just a blend away!

I would love to hear about your smoothie adventures and how this book has inspired your creations. Your feedback and stories are not just valuable to me but also to the community of smoothie enthusiasts we're building together. Please feel free to leave a comment, share your favorite recipe from the book, or suggest new ideas and combinations you've discovered.

Here's to a healthier, happier, and smoother-blending journey!

Your Thoughts Matter!

Your comments and experiences are vital in enriching this journey for all of us. If you've enjoyed the book, found it helpful, or have any suggestions for improvement, please don't hesitate to share your thoughts. Your input will not only inspire future editions of this book but also help fellow readers in their smoothie-making adventures. Let's continue to blend, sip, and share!

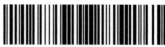